MW00960382

5 Day Pouch Test
Complete Recipe Collection

Find your weight loss surgery tool in five focused days.
LivingAfterWLS Guides Volume 2
(2020 Update 1st Edition)

Kaye Bailey

5 DAY POUCH TEST
COMPLETE RECIPE COLLECTION

FIND YOUR WEIGHT LOSS SURGERY TOOL IN FIVE FOCUSED DAYS.
LIVINGAFTERWLS GUIDES VOLUME 2
(2020 UPDATE 1ST EDITION)

This first edition updated January 30, 2020. This update includes two new feature articles, updated resource links, and 12 new recipes, 24 more pages.

A LIVINGAFTERWLS PUBLICATION
Proudly serving the healthy weight management and
weight loss surgery community since 2005.

COVER © LIVINGAFTERWLS
ADOBE STOCK LICENSED IMAGE BY JENIFOTO

PAPERBACK: ISBN-13: 978-1518844201
COPYRIGHT © LIVINGAFTERWLS
ALL RIGHTS RESERVED

TABLE OF CONTENTS

5 DAY POUCH TEST RECIPES	21
DAYS 1 & 2: LIQUIDS	25
SMOOTHIES & SNACKS	26
SOUPS FOR DAYS 1 & 2	30
READY-MADE SOUPS	33
DAY 3: SOFT PROTEIN	47
EGGS & BAKES	48
BREAKFAST BAKES	51
FISH AND SEAFOOD SOFT PROTEIN	56
QUICK LIST: DIETARY PROTEIN	60
DAY 4: FIRM PROTEIN	63
FISH AND SEAFOOD	63
GROUND MEAT AND POULTRY	73
DAY 5: SOLID PROTEIN	79
DAY 6 RECIPES	91
SMOOTHIES	93
SALADS WITH PROTEIN	103
A WELL-DRESSED SALAD	105
PORK: THE OTHER WHITE MEAT	86
COMPLEX-CARB SIDE DISHES	111
QUICK VEGGIE SIDES	113
RECIPE INDEX	119

NUTRITIONAL ANALYSIS

For purposes of continuity recipe serving size and nutrient values are calculated and measured on the Daily Values standard for a 2,000 calorie per day diet for adults, developed by the Food and Drug Administration (FDA). It is understood that people who have undergone a restrictive bariatric surgical procedure will eat less than the standard serving size, and that people with different bariatric procedures will eat different volumes of food per serving. Please use the serving size and nutrient values provided as the baseline factor from which to calculate and adjust your specific and unique dietary intake.

IMAGINE THE POSSIBILITIES

It seems ironic that our basic need for nutrition, the very fuel that sustains all activities of life and living, is the thing we are least likely to give thought, time, and attention. Imagine what we can accomplish when higher priority is assigned to the preparation and enjoyment of nurturing meals.

Welcome to Your 5 Day Pouch Test Complete Recipe Collection freshly updated for you in 2020 to include: two new feature articles, updated resource links, and 12 new recipes. I think you will appreciate the new menu items and added inspiration as you embark on your 5 Day Pouch Test.

Thank you for joining me in the 5 Day Pouch Test program and making it a valued tool in your weight loss surgery toolbox. In your hands is the 5 Day Pouch Test Complete Recipe Collection. This complete collection of 5 Day Pouch Test triple-tested and approved recipes is a handy companion for getting back to the basics of weight loss surgery using the 5DPT as a tool. You will find over 80 recipes to use on the 5 Day Pouch Test including 28 new recipes beginning on page 77. In addition to recipes there are helpful articles and hints for improving your experience on the 5DPT, ultimately leading you down the path of successful weight management the LivingAfterWLS way.

Who it's for: The 5 Day Pouch Test Complete Recipe Collection is for those who have a modest understanding of the 5DPT plan and wish to have the entire recipe collection at their fingertips, and for people who want to eat well and enjoy long term successful weight management with weight loss surgery.

Stay Connected: Subscribe to the 5 Day Pouch Test Bulletin delivered to your email Inbox. To receive our free monthly digital newsletter, the 5 Day Pouch Test Bulletin, visit 5DayPouchTest.com and enter your email address to subscribe. Also subscribe to our weekly "LivingAfterWLS Digest" and twice-monthly recipe newsletter, "Cooking with Kaye." We value and respect your online information: click the Privacy link on any of our web pages to learn more.

ARE YOU ASKING YOURSELF:

* ✳   Have I lost control of your weight loss surgery tool?
* ✳   Does my pouch still work?
* ✳   Have I broken my pouch?
* ✳   Am I doomed to be a failure at this too?
* ✳   Can I lose the weight I've regained?
* ✳   Is the honeymoon period over?
* ✳   Help! I made goal weight and now I'm gaining.

If you are asking these questions, then the 5 Day Pouch Test is for you. In 5 focused days you can rediscover your pouch, get back on track and lose weight with your weight loss surgery tool. You have not failed. You can learn to use the tool again.

This is the five-day plan that I developed and use to determine if my pouch is working and return to that tight newbie feeling. This plan directly helps one get back to the basics of the weight loss surgery diet and often jump-starts weight loss. It is not difficult to follow and if you are in a stage of snacking and carb-cycling it will break this pattern. Sounds pretty good, right?

Hunger. The 5 Day Pouch Test should never leave you feeling hungry. You can eat as much of the prescribed menu foods as you want during the day to satiate hunger and prevent snacking on slider foods and simple carbohydrates. You must drink a minimum of 64 ounces of water each day. The liquid restrictions (no liquids 30 minutes before or after meals and no liquid with meals) must be observed.

    ✳   5DPT = 5 Day Pouch Test

Weight loss is not the exclusive intent of the 5 Day Pouch Test. However, many who have completed this plan report a pleasing drop in weight. More importantly they celebrate a renewed sense of control over their pouch and eating habits. They easily transition back to a healthy post-surgical weight loss way of eating focused on lean-clean protein, vegetables, fruit, and limited dairy.

Countless thousands of people worldwide have successfully used the 5 Day Pouch Test since 2007 to take control of their weight loss surgery tool. Many have lost regained weight and others are reaching a healthy weight after long stalls in weight loss. But more importantly, feelings of failure are replaced with feelings of empowerment, capability, and personal achievement.

MEAL PLANNING LEADS TO SUCCESS

The people who report the greatest success with the 5DPT and beyond put effort into planning their meals and stick with the plan. It would be easy to provide a very specific 5DPT menu plan, but that takes the opportunity away from plan followers to custom create a meal plan using the concepts provided in the 5DPT. By planning your 5DPT meal plan you get the experience to go beyond the five days and continue making meal plans that support your weight loss surgery goals. This learning experience will serve you well as you pursue life-long weight management maximizing your surgical weight loss tool. Here are a few helpful hints for menu planning:

Learn the plan. Read the plan in full and be sure you understand it. Read the plan completely in order to understand the progression of your diet from Day 1 to Day 5. Pay close attention to understanding the liquid restrictions and slider foods: these are the most common problem areas that lead to weight regain after weight loss surgery. As you become familiar with the 5 Day Pouch Test think back to how it compares with the early dietary stages following your weight loss surgery. Think back to what worked for you then and imagine the same will work for you again. Remember, you already know how to lose weight using your surgical tool. The effort you put into the 5DPT will return you to that place of healthy and reasonable weight management using your tool.

Preparations: Plan your meals for all five days and do the grocery shopping before starting the 5DPT. We all know that the supermarket is temptation alley, do your best to avoid going there for these five days. An effective way to plan your meals is to use the 5 Day Pouch Test menu planner. Make two copies of the 5DPT menu planner and use the first to plan your meals and snacks for all five days. This will become your shopping list as well as your map for the week. Use the second planner to record your actual meals and nutritional consumption. Many people are surprised at the relief and empowerment they feel upon making their food plan for five days. With the menu choices made in advance plan followers are more likely to complete the plan.

✳ Free Download: 5 Day Pouch Test Menu Planner. Visit 5DayPouchTest.com – Click on Tools

Reminder: As you make your menu plan it is perfectly fine to advance food forward over the five days. For example, on Day 3 you may include a serving of soup from Days 1 and 2. On Day 4 include a serving of breakfast bake from Day 3, and so on. This is both an economical and efficient and a strategy to include in your eating plan beyond the 5 Day Pouch Test.

5DPT: BRIEF OVERVIEW

It is only five days. And in the next five days you will learn your pouch is working; you will take control of your eating and snacking behaviors; and you will remember why you had weight loss surgery in the first place.

Days 1 and 2 of the plan are healing days. You treat your pouch like a newborn with gentle liquids and soups. Pouch inflammation is relieved, and processed carbohydrate cravings subside. Mental focus is on listening to and respecting your body. Days 1 and 2 mimic the early days and weeks following bariatric surgery.

Day 3 introduces soft proteins like canned fish, fresh soft fish or eggs. This is the day we focus on tasting our food, chewing well, and enjoying the goodness of lean-clean protein. We focus on portion control and the liquid restrictions. On this day we start to remember what a tight pouch feels like and we appreciate the feeling of fullness.

Day 4 brings us to firm proteins like ground meat (beef, poultry, lamb, or game) and shellfish, scallops, lobster, salmon or halibut steaks. This is the day we truly realize the power of the pouch and most people are happily surprised to learn their pouch is not broken or stretched back to normal stomach size. The carbohydrate withdrawal is over, and energy levels are improving.

Day 5 finishes the test with solid proteins such as white meat poultry, beef steak, and any of the firm proteins from Day 4. The liquid restrictions are now a habit and we have successfully removed the slider foods from our diet. We have energy for exercise and for the daily tasks of living. Most importantly, we know our weight loss surgery tool works and we now have the confidence and capability to work the tool.

Day 6 is the way we will eat every day for the rest of our lives. Having successfully broken a carb-cycle, gained a feeling of control over the surgical gastric pouch, and possibly losing a few pounds one is ready for re-entry into a compliant way of eating. This means focusing on protein dense meals, observing the liquid restrictions, and avoiding starches, particularly processed carbohydrates and slider foods. Three meals a day should be two-thirds protein, one-third healthy carbohydrate in the form of low-glycemic vegetables and fruits. Consumption of whole grains is not forbidden by most centers. However, moderation is necessary and servings of whole grain breads, cereals, and starches must be limited to one serving a day. People who practice this moderation enjoy significantly more weight loss than those who ignore the recommendation.

The following basic tenets are widely accepted by bariatric surgeons and nutritionists as lifestyle guidelines to be followed by people who have undergone all manner of gastric surgery for weight loss. I have found that making these tenets a lifestyle is the most effective way for me and many others to manage weight loss and maintain it with weight loss surgery. Refer to the documentation provided you at the time of your surgery for the specifics advised by your bariatric center.

FOUR RULES: WEIGHT LOSS SURGERY FUNDAMENTALS

At the time of surgery we agreed to follow Four Rules of dietary and lifestyle management guidelines for the rest of our life in order to lose weight and maintain a healthy weight.

All surgical weight loss procedures including gastric bypass, adjustable gastric banding (lap-band) and gastric sleeve, promote weight loss by decreasing energy (caloric) intake with a reduced or restricted stomach size. The small stomach pouch is only effective when a patient rigorously follows the Four Rules: eat a high protein diet; drink lots of water; avoid snacking on empty calorie food; engage in daily exercise.

FOUR RULES:

* ∗   Protein First
* ∗   Lots of Water
* ∗   No Snacking
* ∗   Daily Exercise

Protein First: At every meal the WLS patient will eat lean animal, dairy, or vegetable protein before any other food. Protein shakes or supplements may be included as part of the weight loss surgery diet. Patients are advised to consume 60-105 grams of protein a day. Eating lean protein will create a tight feeling in the surgical stomach pouch: this feeling is the signal to stop eating. Many patients report discomfort when eating lean protein, yet this discomfort is the very reason the stomach pouch is effective in reducing food and caloric intake. Animal products are the most nutrient rich source of protein and include fish, shellfish, poultry, and meat. Dairy protein, including eggs, yogurt, and cheese, is another excellent source of protein.

Lots of Water: Like most weight loss efforts, water consumption for bariatric surgery patient is necessary for weight loss. Most centers advise a minimum of 64 fluid ounces of water each day. Water hydrates the organs and cells and facilitates the metabolic processes of human life. Water flushes toxins and waste from the body. Patients are strongly discouraged from drinking carbonated beverages. In addition, patients are warned against excessive alcohol intake as it tends to have a quicker and more profound intoxicating affect compared with pre-surgery consumption. In addition, non-nutritional beverages of any kind may lead to weight.

No Snacking: Patients are discouraged from snacking which may impede weight loss and lead to weight gain. Specifically, patients are forbidden to partake of traditional processed carbohydrate snacks, such as chips, crackers, baked goods, and sweets. Patients who return to snacking on empty calorie non-nutritional food defeat the restrictive nature of the surgery and weight gain results. It is seemingly contradictory that the 5DPT allows snacking. High protein snacks are allowed because they keep the metabolism active, they satiate hunger, and they help relieve the symptoms of carbohydrate withdrawal.

Daily Exercise: In general patients are advised to engage in 30 minutes of physical activity on most days of the week. The most effective way to heal the body from the ravages of obesity is to exercise. Exercise means moving the body: walking, stretching, bending, inhaling and exhaling. Exercise is the most effective, most enjoyable, most beneficial gift one can receive when recovering from life threatening, crippling morbid obesity. Consistent exercise will keep morbid obesity in remission and help compensate for lapses in following the three other rules. People who successfully maintain their weight exercise daily.

SLIDER FOOD & LIQUID RULES

Slider Foods: To the weight loss surgery patient slider foods are the bane of good intentions often causing dumping syndrome, weight loss plateaus, and eventually weight gain. As defined, slider foods are soft simple processed carbohydrates of little or no nutritional value that slide right through the surgical stomach pouch without providing nutrition or satiation. The most commonly consumed slider foods include pretzels, crackers (saltines, graham, Ritz®, etc.) filled cracker snacks such as Ritz Bits®, popcorn, cheese snacks (Cheetos®) or cheese crackers, tortilla chips with salsa, potato chips, sugar-free cookies, cakes, and candy.

The very nature of the surgical gastric pouch is to cause feelings of tightness or restriction when one has eaten enough food. However, when soft simple carbohydrates are eaten this tightness or restriction does not result and one can continue to eat, unmeasured amounts of food without ever feeling uncomfortable. Many patients unknowingly turn to slider foods for this very reason. They do not like the discomfort that results when the pouch is full, the result of eating a measured portion of lean animal or dairy protein, and it is more comfortable to eat the soft slider foods.

Liquid Restrictions: After surgical weight loss patients are advised to avoid drinking liquids 30 minutes before meals and 30 minutes after meals. (The time restriction varies from surgeon to surgeon, but most use the 30 minutes before, 30 minutes after restriction. Follow your surgeon's specific directions.) Additionally, there should be no liquid consumed while eating. Following these liquid restrictions allows the pouch to feel tight sooner and stay tight longer, thus leaving the patient feeling satiated for greater periods of time without experiencing the urge to snack.

One thing often overlooked is that following the time or liquid restrictions allows the small stomach time to digest and allocate the nutrients including vitamins and minerals in your food. After surgery we have less stomach in which nutrient breakdown and absorption may occur. The liquid restrictions allow the intestine to function efficiently thus improving your overall health and wellness. Called metabolism, we know this process is boosted by the high protein diet and we lose more weight, without doing much more than respect the guideline.

Learn a great deal more about the metabolism boosting power of the high protein diet in our LivingAfterWLS Guide Volume 3: Protein First: Understanding and Living the First Rule of Weight Loss Surgery. Available online in digital and paperback.

We can give all the attention in the world to well-planned protein first meals. But if we chew, swallow, and wash-it down the effort is wasted. In addition, the longer food stays in the small gastric pouch the more opportunity the body must absorb nutrients from that food. The liquid restrictions should be followed when eating all meals and snacks, including protein shakes, protein bars, hearty soups, and solid protein main dishes.

Plan your 5DPT Menu

One of the best ways to enable your success with the 5 Day Pouch Advance planning your meals for the duration of the plan will increase the likelihood of sticking with the plan and enjoying success as you march forward. This is not a difficult task as you are only planning for five days. Many find having a complete plan to be liberating: the decision making is done. One must only concentrate on following the plan and focusing on surgical pouch and how it functions when used properly. Here are some helpful suggestions for planning your 5DPT menu:

Plan three meals (breakfast, lunch, dinner) and two or three 5DPT snacks. Foods from Days 1 and 2 may be advanced to Days 3, 4, and 5. Do not have Day 3, 4, and 5 food before the intended day.

Purchase ingredients before beginning Day 1 and avoid going to the market during the five days. The 5DPT will help build your resistance to marketing temptation, but during the five days the temptation may simply be an annoying distraction.

If you haven't tried protein gelatin or protein pudding before you begin the plan, please make a sample before Day 1. Make certain that what you plan is something you will enjoy eating. Consider 1-cup servings of soup as a suitable snack on any day of the 5DPT.

If including soups on Days 1 and 2 prepare them in advance before Day 1 and divide into 1-cup serving containers for ease of use.

The 5DPT recipes are healthy and family friendly. Try to include the people at your table in your menu and avoid cooking two meals. For others add vegetables, a salad or a starch as desired.

16

Try to stick with your menu plan as closely as possible. Sometimes change is unavoidable. Do the best you can at each meal staying as close to your plan as possible.

SAMPLE 5 DAY POUCH TEST MENU

DAY 1:

- Breakfast: Choco-Mocha Morning Smoothie
- Morning Snack: High-Protein Gelatin
- Lunch: Vanilla-Berry Smoothie
- Afternoon Snack: 1/2 apple
- Dinner: 1 cup 5DPT soup of your Choice
- Evening Snack: High Protein Pudding

DAY 2:

- Breakfast: Choco-Mocha Morning Smoothie
- Morning Snack: Frozen Protein Pudding Pop
- Lunch: 1 cup 5DPT soup of your choice
- Afternoon Snack: High Protein Gelatin
- Dinner: 1 cup 5DPT soup of your Choice
- Evening Snack: High Protein Pudding

DAY 3:

- Breakfast: Mock Breakfast Burrito
- Morning Snack: High Protein Gelatin
- Lunch: Parmesan Tuna Patty
- Afternoon Snack: Frozen Protein Pudding Pop
- Dinner: Parmesan Tuna Patty
- Evening Snack: High Protein Gelatin

17

DAY 4:

- Breakfast: Spinach-Sausage Egg Bake
- Morning Snack: 1 small orange
- Lunch: Parmesan Tuna Patty (leftover from Day 3)
- Afternoon Snack: 1 small pear and 1/2 cup cottage cheese
- Dinner: Orange Glazed Salmon
- Evening Snack: High Protein Pudding

DAY 5:

- Breakfast: Egg Brunch Bake
- Morning Snack: 1 piece of low-glycemic fruit
- Lunch: Orange Glazed Salmon (leftover from Day 4)
- Afternoon Snack: High Protein Gelatin
- Dinner: Chicken and Pea Pods
- Evening Snack: Frozen Protein Pudding Pop

✳ *Meal Planner: You can download this worksheet, and all worksheets for free at 5DayPouchTest.com.   Click Downloads. LivingAfterWLS recently introduced a new line of life planners bespoke for the weight loss surgery patient. They address our special dietary and health management needs and focus on the long journey, not just a quick trip to goal weight. Stay on track! These planners are terrific tools to keep us on point. Find them exclusively on Amazon in print format. See my author page for a current catalog of all our publications. Kaye Bailey Amazon Page*

WEEK OF: _____

MEAL PLANNER

MONDAY

TUESDAY

WEDNESDAY

THURSDAY

FRIDAY

SATURDAY

SUNDAY

SHOPPING LIST:

WEEK OF: MEAL PLANNER

MONDAY

SHOPPING LIST:

TUESDAY

WEDNESDAY

THURSDAY

FRIDAY

SATURDAY

SUNDAY

5 DAY POUCH TEST RECIPES

Here you will find all the recipes you need for a delicious and successful 5 Day Pouch Test. These recipes have been tested time and again for their effectiveness in the 5DPT and your gratification both during the plan and for many meals beyond. In addition to enjoying these recipes use them as guides to model your own favorite meals balancing lean protein prepared with fresh healthful complex carbohydrates and controlled amounts of healthy fat.

Avoid substitutions: During the 5DPT please avoid substitutions as much as possible. Each recipe is designed specifically for the designated day of the plan with the amount of protein, carbohydrate, and fat it contains. Changes may decrease the effectiveness of your plan.

Nutritional Analysis: Every effort has been made to check the accuracy of the nutritional information that appears with each recipe. However, because numerous variables account for a wide range of values for certain foods, nutritive analyses in this book should be considered approximate. Different results may be obtained by using different nutrient databases and different brand-name products.

Before you start: Tame a Grumpy Pouch

Do you have a grumpy pouch? Here is a healing soup to ease your pouchy woes. We sometimes turn to the 5 Day Pouch Test when we have been eating all the wrong things and we have an inflamed digestive system; sometimes we call this a grumpy pouch. If you are feeling particularly poorly going into the 5DPT consider making this soup the day before and enjoy the healing benefits of the ingredients that are natural digestive aids. This recipe is a great remedy any time you experience a grumpy pouch, use it even when you are not following the 5 Day Pouch Test.

Fennel and celery are both good digestive healers. Fennel is known to soothe an inflamed digestive lining and celery helps to support liver function. Raw vegetables can irritate an inflamed digestive system, so this well-cooked soup soothes the digestive system and helps cleanse your body of toxins. Feel free to enjoy a 1-cup serving as a snack on any day of the 5DPT. Remember to observe the liquid restrictions, especially when eating soup. You want to make sure your body has time to absorb and digest the wholesome nutrients that come from a carefully made soup.

Fennel and Celery "Grumpy Pouch" Soup

    1 large white or yellow onion, chopped (about 1 cup)
    2 bulbs of root fennel, peeled and chopped
    8 ribs of celery, chopped
    4 cups vegetable stock, reduced sodium
    2 bay leaves
    1 tablespoon fresh parsley, finely chopped

Parsley sprigs for garnish

Directions: Place all of the ingredients in a large saucepan and bring to a boil. Reduce to a low boil and cook for 10 minutes. Further reduce temperature to a slow simmer and cook an additional 30 minutes. Remove from heat and allow cooling. Remove and discard the bay leaves. Using a blender or immersion blender puree the soup until smooth. Return to saucepan and gently reheat. Thin the soup to desired consistency with additional vegetable broth. Enjoy a 1-cup serving of soup as needed to relieve a distressed stomach. Store refrigerated 3 to 4 days.

WARM LEMON WATER

Drink warm lemon water. Warm lemon water is an energy booster; provides hydrating electrolytes in the form of potassium, calcium and magnesium; reduces inflammation; improves digestion; helps regulate bowel movements; strengthens immune system; improves mood while reducing depression and anxiety associated with potassium deficiency; and improves weight loss by suppressing hunger cravings. Is it any wonder that cleanse programs prescribe warm lemon water first thing each day?

Warm Lemon Water is easy to prepare. Add 8 ounces warm (not boiling) water to a mug, add 1-2 tablespoons 100% pure lemon juice* and sweeten as desired with honey, agave syrup, or preferred beverage sweetener. Drink warm.

✳ *I use ReaLemon 100% Juice from concentrate most of the time. While freshly squeezed lemon juice is delightful it takes an extra step in squeezing the juice vs. a quick pour from the bottle. At times fresh juicing is an inconvenient barrier. The juice concentrate removes the barrier and the excuse. Do what works for you!*

CONSTIPATION AND THE 5 DAY POUCH TEST?

HERE ARE SOME SUGGESTIONS:

- Eat 1/2 apple with skin for your mid-morning and mid-afternoon snack
- Increase your fluid intake
- Include a water-soluble fiber supplement in your daily diet
- Add a fish oil capsule to your diet
- Drink herbal tea containing senna leaf in a small portion (6 fluid ounces): it is a powerful natural laxative.
- Prepare one of the Feed the Carb Monster Soups for days 1 & 2 (each 1-cup serving contains 5 grams dietary fiber). Look on the Internet 5daypouchtest.com or in the 5 Day Pouch Test Owner's Manual for recipes.

DAYS 1 & 2: LIQUIDS

Days 1 and 2 of the plan are healing days. You treat your pouch like a newborn with gentle protein fortified liquids and soups. Pouch inflammation is reduced, and processed carbohydrate cravings subside. Mental focus is on listening to and respecting your body. Your menu on Days 1 and 2 repeats the early days and weeks following bariatric surgery. A diet of simple liquids, including protein drinks, clear broth, creamy soups, and hearty soups takes the guess work out of meal planning so you can focus on making well your WLS tool.

All meals on Days 1 and 2 are liquids as defined here. In the 5 Day Pouch Test liquids are defined to include clear broth and creamy soups, protein fortified beverages (protein shakes/smoothies), and hearty soups made of vegetables, legumes with some animal protein and dairy. Plan your days to include some of these healthful recipes that have been tested and found effective

* *Gentle Reminder: Coffee is coffee. Water is water. Coffee is a diuretic and will slow weight loss. Water will flush toxins and waste from your body and facilitate weight loss.*

SMOOTHIES & SNACKS

These smoothie recipes call for protein powder. They also go by the name protein shakes or protein liquid meal replacement. More importantly, they are fresh and refreshing—whatever you call them. Easy to prepare they are flavor packed and satiating. I use a variety of protein powders chosen because they provide 20 grams of high-quality whey protein isolate per serving and are palatable.

High-quality whey protein isolate is often labeled medical grade which means it is approved for use in a clinical setting where a patient's nutritional intake is managed by medical staff (hospital, elder care, long-term illness care., etc.). You can order medical quality protein products online. Recent attention to low-carb dieting for weight loss has prompted growth in the engineered protein consumer food products. It may take some experimenting to find a product that appeals to your taste and meets your nutritional requirements. The effort it takes to find a product you will use is worth it. Protein supplements can only work if we use them. Simple, right?

Are you enjoying DaVinci Gourmet Sugar Free Syrups? I use them to enhance the flavor in my smoothies. You can find them in stores and online davincigourmet.com.

CHOCO-MOCHA MORNING SMOOTHIE

1 scoop chocolate flavored protein powder
1 cup skim milk or SOYMILK

1 tablespoon of decaf instant coffee granules

1 tablespoon DaVinci chocolate sugar free syrup

Directions: Place all ingredients in the blender and blend until smooth and foamy. Hint: If you like an iced smoothie, make ice cubes from brewed coffee and add them to the ingredients as desired. Nutritionals are product-variable: refer to product label to estimate nutritional values.

∗ *Adjust the sweetness to your taste using the no-calorie sweetener of your choice.*

VANILLA-BERRY SMOOTHIE

½ cup vanilla low-fat yogurt

1 cup skim milk or SOYMILK

1 scoop vanilla protein powder

½ cup frozen berries

Directions: Place all ingredients in the blender and blend until smooth and foamy. Hint: Fresh fruit may be used in place of frozen and will help reduce the headache that may result from carbohydrate withdrawal. Nutritionals will vary depending upon ingredients and products used. Refer to product label to estimate nutritional values.

STRAWBERRIES & WHITE CHOCOLATE SMOOTHIE

1 cup of water, chilled

1 scoop Strawberry flavor protein powder

½ cup frozen strawberries

1 tablespoon DaVinci White Chocolate Sugar Free Syrup

Directions: Place all ingredients in the blender and blend until smooth and frothy. Serve in a chilled glass. Nutritionals will vary depending upon ingredients and products used. Refer to product label to estimate nutritional values. Serving Hint: treat yourself to a beautifully presented meal, you deserve it. A well-presented meal enhances the eating experience and is believed to contribute to prolonged satiety following a meal.

HIGH PROTEIN PUDDING

Package high protein pudding in single serving containers to grab when a quick snack is required to boost energy and stave off hunger. For on the go meals transport pudding in a cooled lunchbox and serve chilled.

2 cups cold skim milk or SOYMILK
2 scoops unflavored protein powder
1 (4-servings) package sugar free instant pudding, any flavor

Directions: In a 2-quart bowl whisk together the cold milk and the protein powder. Whisk in the instant pudding mix, cover and chill. Nutrition: Serves 4. Per ½-cup serving: 145 calories, 14 grams protein, 2 grams fat, trace carbohydrate.

FROZEN PROTEIN PUDDING POPS

These frozen pudding pops are a refreshing treat that can be enjoyed, in moderation, during the 5DPT and the days to follow. Always remember to follow the liquid restrictions when enjoying these treats for a snack or mini meal.

2 (11-ounce) ready-to-drink protein drinks, flavor of your choice
1 (4-servings) package sugar-free pudding mix

Directions: In a medium bowl whisk together protein drinks and pudding mix. Divide evenly in ice pop molds or small paper cups with wooden sticks or spoons inserted in pudding mix. Freeze until solid. Serve frozen. Note: Nutritional information varies by ingredients.

HIGH PROTEIN GELATIN

This is the recipe commonly prepared in hospitals for patients recovering from gastric and intestinal surgeries. Many WLS patients continue to include this health-promoting mini-meal in their diet long after healing from surgery.

1 (4 servings) package sugar free gelatin, any flavor
1/3 cup dried (powdered) egg whites
boiling water and cold water per package directions

Directions: Prepare the sugar-free gelatin according to package directions. When gelatin is dissolved, and cold water has been added whisk-in powdered egg whites until completely dissolved. Do not substitute liquid egg whites. Chill until set. Serve cold. For a treat add a 1-tablespoon dollop of fat-free, sugar free non-dairy topping. Nutrition: 4 servings. Per serving: 35 calories, 9 grams protein.

BONUS BENEFIT FROM GELATIN:

It has long been known that gelatin supports nail and hair growth and that's not just beauty shop gossip. Blame it on those amino acids again! Nails and hair are composed of protein and the amino acids in gelatin provide the building blocks to make them stronger, grow more quickly and reflect your good health with bounce and shine. Adding gelatin to your diet during the first year following weight loss surgery may help to lessen the loss of hair reported by so many bariatric patients. Gelatin is on the approved foods list for all post-surgery dietary stages so give it a chance to love you back. Vegetarians can find plant-based gelatin made of red algae in health food stores.

SOUPS FOR DAYS 1 & 2

Featured here are soup recipes that can be used as your liquid meals for Days 1 and 2 of the 5DPT. Feedback from plan testers suggests that liquids, such as broth or protein shakes, for some are not satiating and some are struggling to get past the first two days of liquids on the 5DPT. These soups meet the protein requirement, the liquid requirement and they include enough fat and carbohydrate to fuel your body during the pouch test leaving you energized and satiated. In addition, these recipes will help regulate your metabolic hormones -insulin and glucagon- which may be out of balance if you are endeavoring to correct a simple-carb snacking habit.

You will notice these recipes are slightly higher in fat than our typical recipes from LivingAfterWLS. Humans need dietary fat and use it efficiently as fuel. When fat is ingested without being wrapped in white carbohydrates, we tend to be self-regulating with our fat intake. Have you ever sat down to eat a stick of butter or drink a cup of olive oil? Quite unappealing. When snack foods -chips, French fries, doughnuts, cakes, pies, pastries and such- are eliminated from the diet the body adjusts to lower fat intake and cravings diminish.

Follow the directions closely: not all soups need to be pureed or blended until smooth. When serving and enjoying soups the most important step is to measure portions, never exceeding 1 cup per serving.

HAM & CHEESE SOUP

This is a rich creamy soup that pairs the classic flavors of ham and cheese for a delicious meal in a bowl.

2 tablespoons butter
½ cup carrots, chopped
¼ cup onion, chopped
2 tablespoons flour
1 teaspoon paprika
1 teaspoon dry mustard
6 cups chicken broth, reduced sodium
1 (12-ounce) package processed cheese spread (Velveeta®), reduced-fat, shredded
1 (12-ounce) package light firm silken tofu, diced
2 (5-ounce) cans deviled ham spread
1 cup sour cream, low-fat
salt and pepper, to taste
¼ cup Parmesan cheese, grated
parsley sprigs, for garnish

Directions: In a large Dutch oven over medium heat melt butter. Add carrots and onion and cook and stir until soft and translucent. Stir in flour, paprika and dry mustard using a whisk. Cook for 2 minutes then slowly add the chicken broth whisking to prevent lumps. When soup is thickened add shredded Velveeta®, the diced tofu and ham. Simmer for 20 minutes stirring occasionally. Remove from heat and stir in sour cream. Add salt and pepper to taste and serve garnished with a sprinkle of Parmesan cheese and a sprig of parsley. Nutrition: Serves: 10. Per 1-cup serving: 264 calories, 19 grams protein, 15 grams fat and 12 grams carbohydrate.

✳ *Note: Substituting reduced-fat cheese in place of the processed cheese spread may result in a lumpy mixture. Instead, try reduced-fat cream cheese if you prefer it to processed cheese. Don't eliminate the tofu as this vegetarian high protein ingredient is essential to nutritional completeness.*

GOOD HABIT: MEASURE SOUP

What I've learned is that soups must be measured. Clear soups or smooth soups without solids should be measured in 1-cup servings and eaten within about 15 minutes. Soups and stews with solids must also be measured, but differently. Use a slotted spoon scoop out solids into a 1/2-cup measuring cup. Put that in your bowl, and then add an additional 1/2-cup of the soup - both liquid and solids. This makes a good hearty 1-cup serving that should keep us full and satiated for a long time after the meal. Thick chili with beans and meat is best measured in 2/3-cup servings. It seems like these hearty dishes are much more filling: it is best to start with a smaller portion. Again, with hearty chili and stews avoid eating more than 1-cup volume for any meal.

LOW-CARB PUMPKIN & SAUSAGE SOUP

This is a universal favorite soup. In place of the pumpkin use a butternut squash puree if you prefer. Canned pumpkin puree is nearly as nutritious as raw pumpkin containing vitamin A, beta carotene and dietary fiber.

1 (16-ounce) package country style sausage
1 small onion, minced (about ½ cup)
1 clove garlic, minced

1 tablespoon Italian seasoning

1 cup fresh mushrooms, chopped

1 (15-ounce) can 100% pure pumpkin

5 cups chicken broth, reduced sodium

½ cup heavy cream

½ cup sour cream

½ cup water

Directions: Over medium heat cook the sausage breaking into small bits. Drain fat. Add the onion, garlic, Italian seasoning, and mushrooms, and cook and stir until vegetables are tender. Add the canned pumpkin, and the broth, stirring well. Cook at a low simmer for 20 to 30 minutes. Remove from heat and stir in heavy cream, sour cream, and water. Serve warm. This soup freezes well in single-serving portions. This soup should not be pureed. Nutrition: Serves 8. Per 1-cup serving: 376 calories, 15 grams protein, 32 grams fat, 9 grams carbohydrate.

✳   *Ingredient Note: Country style sausage is bulk ground sausage not in casings. Jimmy Dean® Premium Pork Mild Country Sausage, also called roll sausage, is a nationally available country style sausage that works very well in this recipe.*

READY-MADE SOUPS

Campbell's Healthy Request® Cream of Mushroom Soup is a good commercial soup that works well on the 5DPT. A 1-cup serving of soup prepared with 2% milk provides 130 calories, 6 grams protein, 5 grams fat (1 gram saturated), 10 grams carbohydrate.

For on-the-go meals try Campbell's Soup at Hand® 25% Less Sodium Classic Tomato Soup. Heated quickly in the microwave and served in the same container this convenient soup provides 140 calories, 3 grams protein, 0 grams fat, 33 grams. Use these examples to find nutritionally compatible ready-to-eat soups to include in your 5DPT and beyond.

PUMPKIN SHRIMP SOUP

This is another delicious pumpkin soup you will enjoy on Days 1 and 2. Consider stocking-up on canned pumpkin during the fall and winter seasons when it is readily available and priced reasonably. Canned pumpkin can sometimes be difficult to find during the spring and summer.

2 tablespoons unsalted butter
2 medium onions, sliced
2 medium carrots, sliced
2 medium garlic cloves, minced
1 teaspoon Old Bay Seafood Seasoning®
1 (14-ounce) can fat free reduced sodium chicken broth
1 (15-ounce) can pumpkin puree, no added salt
1 cup whole milk or 1 cup reduced fat evaporated milk
8 ounces cooked shrimp, peeled and deveined (if frozen, thawed)
freshly grated nutmeg for garnish, optional

Directions: Over medium-high heat in a large soup pot, melt butter and cook the onions, carrots, and garlic, covered until tender, about 10-12 minutes, stirring occasionally. Stir in the Old Bay Seafood Seasoning® and half of the chicken broth. Working in batches puree the cooked vegetables in a blender or food processor following safety guidelines for processing hot food (see article below). Return vegetable puree to cooking pot. Alternatively, use an immersion blender to puree the soup directly in the pot.

To vegetable puree add the remaining broth, pumpkin puree, milk, and thawed drained shrimp. Heat gently to a low simmer, not boiling, continue cooking 5 minutes until soup thickens slightly and is warm throughout. Serve immediately in measured 1 cup portions. Garnish each serving with a sprinkle of freshly grated nutmeg. Nutrition: Serves 6. Per 1 cup serving: 245 calories, 19 grams protein, 5 grams fat, 23 grams carbohydrate, 6 grams dietary fiber.

✳ *Cooking Hint: For leftovers reheat in the microwave on medium power to avoid overcooking the shrimp.*

✳ *Ingredient Substitutions: Canned shrimp, crabmeat, or salmon would work equally well in place of the frozen shrimp. Be certain you have 8-ounces of seafood solids after draining the liquid. Label weight often includes water weight in canned fish and seafood.*

SAFELY BLEND HOT LIQUIDS

Using the blender to puree soup is a good method for getting a smooth soup providing certain precautions are followed. Never fill the blender more than half-way and use warm liquids that are well below the boiling point. Most blenders come with a removable stopper on the lid. When blending hot liquids this stopper must be removed and a folded towel can be held in place over the stopper hole. If the stopper is in place steam from the hot liquid creates pressure that literally blasts off the lid creating danger and causing a mess. Blend the mixture with pulses until the desired consistency is reached. Rewarm the pureed soup in the cooking pot.

LEMONY CHICKEN SOUP

I found this recipe in Prevention Best Weight Loss Recipes and was intrigued with the inclusion of two eggs at the end of cooking. This method is like egg drop soup, but I had never considered adding an egg to a hearty soup. Have you? The result is a fresh and light chicken soup with a creamy texture thanks to the addition of eggs. Each 1-cup serving provides 25 grams protein. This soup works well in the 5 Day Pouch Test and will become a Day 6 favorite as well.

1 teaspoon olive oil
1 small clove garlic, minced
6 cups chicken broth, reduced sodium
1 rib celery, chopped
1 cup shredded carrots
½ teaspoon ground black pepper
¼ teaspoon salt
½ cup orzo* (small-grain pasta)
2½ cups frozen green peas or green beans
3 cups chopped cooked chicken
2 large eggs
3-4 tablespoons freshly squeezed lemon juice (about 1 large lemon)

Directions: Heat olive oil in a Dutch oven over medium heat. Add garlic and cook until light brown, about 1 minute. Add broth, celery, carrots, pepper, and salt and bring to a boil over high heat. Add orzo and reduce heat to a simmer. Cook until orzo is tender, about 8 minutes. Add peas and chicken and simmer 2 minutes. (Preparation Note: If freezing portions of this soup do so at this step, before adding eggs. Add eggs to thawed soup in final stage of reheating.) Meanwhile whisk eggs and 3 tablespoons of the lemon juice in medium bowl. Temper egg mixture by slowly whisking in about 1 cup hot broth in a thin stream. Whisk egg mixture into soup and warm briefly over low heat, 2 minutes. Do not boil or eggs will curdle. Adjust seasoning to taste with lemon juice, salt, and pepper and serve. Nutrition: Serves 6. Per 1 cup serving: 212 calories, 25 grams protein, 5 grams fat, 16 grams carbohydrate (2 grams dietary fiber).

✳ *Ingredient Note: In Italian orzo means barley, but it's actually tiny, rice-shaped pasta, slightly smaller than a pine nut. Orzo is ideal for soups and wonderful when served as a substitute for rice. Look for orzo in the pasta aisle.*

TOMATO-CHICKPEA SOUP: VEGETARIAN

One question I answer often is "Can I have tomato soup on the 5DPT?" Most tomato soups are heavy with fat and slight on the protein content. However, I recently came across this recipe for Tomato Chickpea Soup and it works well for Days 1 and 2 of the Pouch Test and can also be included in a healthy Day 6 and beyond menu. Not only are the chickpeas nutritionally dense, they are filling and add healthy vegetable protein to the dish. This soup does not have the familiar rich cream texture of traditional soup, but I think you find it quite satisfying. Remember, a serving size is 1 cup. This recipe makes 6 cups so you will have leftovers to enjoy for meals later in the week.

3 garlic cloves, minced
½ teaspoon
pinch red-pepper chili flakes
1 teaspoon ground coriander
3/4 teaspoon coarse salt
1/8 teaspoon caraway seeds
2 tablespoons extra-virgin olive oil

1 (15-ounce) can chickpeas, drained and rinsed
1 (15-ounce) can crushed tomatoes, reduced sodium
3½ cups homemade or reduced sodium chicken stock
sour cream for topping

Directions: Using a mortar and pestle or the back of a spoon, crush garlic, chili flakes, coriander, salt, and caraway to form a paste. In a heavy 2-quart saucepan over medium-high heat, heat oil. Add garlic and chili mixture, and cook until just softened, about 3 minutes. Stir in chickpeas, tomatoes, roasted red peppers, and stock. Simmer, stirring often, for 15 minutes. Let cool slightly. Working in batches, puree soup in a blender or use an immersion blender. Rewarm if necessary. Serve with a dollop of sour cream if desired. Nutrition: Serves 6. Per 1-cup serving and 1 teaspoon sour cream: 173 calories, 11 grams protein, 8 grams fat (1 saturated), 22 grams carbohydrate.

✳ *Ingredient Note: for variety try different canned tomatoes including those flavored with roasted garlic, olive oil, or roasted peppers.*

SOUP ON THE GO:

There are times when we will need to eat restaurant food during the 5 Day Pouch Test and on Day 6 and beyond. A carefully selected soup can be a favorable choice on the menu. Review these restaurant choices and look at their nutritional score. You can find many restaurant menus online and they often contain nutritional values.

On the menu look for: 1-cup soup servings with 8-21 grams protein; low-glycemic vegetables, beans and legumes that provide nutrient rich complex carbohydrates and dietary fiber; avoid all trans-fat; Sodium should be 1,000mg or lower. Soups made with fresh seasonal vegetables are always a good choice.

Panera Bread Low-Fat Vegetarian Black Bean Soup: A 1-cup serving provides 150 calories and 8 grams protein. That is a little low for protein requirements per meal, but the soup also provides 6 grams of fiber while being low in fat and virtually trans-fat free. The carbs, measuring 28 grams per serving, seem high at first glance. But black beans are low-glycemic (GI Value 30) complex carbohydrates. Black beans are an ideal food for fighting carb cravings. They are rich in folate, manganese, thiamin (B vitamins) and potassium

✳ *When selecting soup pay attention to the ingredient lists and nutrition information provided by the restaurant. Look for a short list of ingredients with recognizable names, meaning the item is made with few additives and preservatives.*

Wendy's Cup of Chili: A small serving of Wendy's Chili (about 1 cup) provides 190 calories with 14 grams protein, 5 grams fiber, 19 grams carbohydrate (again - low GI), and is low in fat. The sodium comes in high at 830mg in this serving size. That is 36% of the recommended sodium intake of 2,300mg/day. Enjoy this tasty cup of chili in moderation and seek lower sodium food choices for other meals consumed that day.

Boston Market Chicken Noodle Soup: A 6-ounce serving provides 170 calories with 13 grams protein and 17 grams carbohydrate. Like most commercially prepared soups the sodium is high at 930mg per serving, 38% of your daily value. This is a broth-based soup. That means it is very important to remember the liquid restrictions and avoid drinking fluids for 30 minutes before and 30 minutes after eating. This will help your pouch stay full longer and give your body a better opportunity to absorb the nutrients. One benefit of eating soups when dining out is that your mouth stays moist making conversation more pleasant without the inclusion of additional liquids during the meal.

THE JOY OF SOUP

It is not very often that I hear from someone who struggles with technical issues when eating soup after weight loss surgery. Soup doesn't get "stuck" going down and if we eat too much the discomfort is short-lived (compared to eating too much solid food that is poorly chewed and eaten quickly). In fact, when post-WLS patients discover soup it often becomes their go-to comfort food. When animal protein is cooked into a soup it is moist and succulent making it easy to chew, swallow, and digest. Cooked vegetables are agreeably tolerated by many WLS-ers compared to raw vegetables. And grains like pearl barley or quinoa are portion controlled and digestible when included as an ingredient in soup. Perhaps it sounds cliché but there is truly joy in a simple healthy cup of soup.

Stock your freezer: Soups, stocks, and broths are easy to freeze. Use heavy-duty freezer bags or plastic containers but be sure to leave some room for expansion as the liquids freeze. Label containers with contents and date and be sure to mark down a use-by date (in general, three months). Freshly prepared broth or stock can be frozen in ice cube trays and used in recipes by adding the frozen cube of stock directly to the cooking pot.

CREAM OF TURKEY SOUP

This is a quick and healthy way to use leftover Thanksgiving turkey. Leftover chicken or shredded rotisserie chicken is also good in place of the turkey.

4 tablespoons (½ stick) unsalted butter
1 large onion, chopped
10 ounces cooked turkey, finely shredded (discard skin)
2½ cups chicken stock
1 tablespoon fresh tarragon
½ cup heavy cream

Directions: Melt the butter in a large, heavy bottom pan, then add the onion and cook for 3 minutes. Add the turkey to the pan with 1½ cups of the chicken stock. Bring to a boil, then let simmer for 20 minutes. Remove the pan from the heat and let cool. Transfer the soup to a food processor or blender and process until smooth. Add the remainder of the stock and season to taste with salt and pepper. Garnish with the tarragon and add a swirl of heavy cream. Serve warm. Nutrition: Serves 4. Per serving: 342 calories, 18 grams protein, 28 grams fat, 4 grams carbohydrate.

HAM & SPLIT PEA SOUP

Split peas are a widely popular legume available year-round throughout the United States. They are an abundant source of fiber and protein and supply a goodly amount of minerals including potassium, and the disease fighting B-vitamin, folate. A mild sausage compliments the flavor of split pea soup, but for a spicier soup select a hot sausage. Consider garnishing with sour cream to add richness and dairy protein.

8 slices bacon or 8 ounces bulk pork sausage
½ medium white or yellow onion, chopped
1 cup carrot, chopped
1-pound dry green split peas
16 ounces chicken broth
2 cups water
1 cup ham cubes
1 each bay leaf
ground pepper, to taste
¼ teaspoon nutmeg, freshly grated

Directions: In a large heavy Dutch oven cook the bacon or sausage over moderate heat, stirring until crisp. Transfer to paper towels to drain. Leave rendered bacon fat in pot and cook the onion and carrots until translucent and soft. Add remaining ingredients and bring to a simmer. Simmer uncovered, stirring occasionally for two hours. Add more water if soup is too thick for your taste. The soup should be dense in order to leave you feeling full longer. Discard bay leaf and serve warm topped with crumbled bacon. Nutrition: Serves: 12. Per 1-cup serving: 184 calories; 13 grams protein, 4 grams fat, 25 grams carbohydrate, 10 grams dietary fiber.

DEFINING VEGETARIAN

For our purposes with the 5DPT some recipes are sub-titled vegetarian. These are lacto-ovo vegetarian recipes. According to Suzanne Havala, M.S., R.D. in Being Vegetarian for Dummies, "A *lacto-ovo vegetarian diet excludes meat, fish, and poultry but includes dairy products and eggs. Most vegetarians in the U.S., Canada, and Western Europe fall into this category. Lacto-ovo vegetarians eat such foods as cheese, ice cream, yogurt, milk, and eggs, as well as foods made with these ingredients."* Please reference this definition when selecting recipes from LivingAfterWLS publications to support a vegetarian diet.

BLACK BEAN SOUP: VEGETARIAN

Beans are naturally a low-glycemic food and one of nature's nutritional power packs. They are considered good sources of protein, fiber, B vitamins, iron, zinc and magnesium.

1 cup dry black beans
olive oil spray
½ cup diced onion
½ cup diced celery
½ cup diced carrot
1 large red pepper, roasted
1 tablespoon minced fresh garlic
2 quarts vegetable broth
¼ teaspoon ground cumin
½ teaspoon salt
1 teaspoon chopped fresh oregano
2 teaspoons chopped fresh parsley
2 teaspoons chopped fresh cilantro

Directions: In a large bowl, cover black beans with 4 cups of water and soak overnight. Rinse beans in a colander with fresh water and drain. Lightly spray a large saucepan with olive oil spray. Over medium-high heat cook and stir onion, celery, carrot, roasted pepper, and garlic Add vegetable broth and black beans. Bring to a boil, reduce heat, and simmer for 1 hour. When beans are tender, pour into a food processor and puree. Add cumin, salt, oregano, parsley, and cilantro. Nutrition: Serves 6. Per 1-cup serving: 140 calories, 13 grams protein, 27 grams carbohydrate, 5 grams dietary fiber.

LENTIL & BARLEY SOUP: VEGETARIAN

Both lentils and barely are low-glycemic, and each ingredient has a hearty distinctive flavor, contributing to this zesty, satisfying winter soup: a complete meal in a bowl. The turmeric and curry powder lend an exotic flavor.

1 tablespoon oil
1 large onion, finely chopped
2 cloves garlic, crushed or 2 teaspoons minced garlic
½ teaspoon turmeric
2 teaspoons curry powder
½ teaspoon ground cumin
1 teaspoon red pepper flakes
6 cups water
1½ cups vegetable or chicken stock
1 cup red lentils
½ cup pearl barley
1 (15-ounce) can crushed tomatoes
salt and pepper to taste
fresh parsley, chopped, for garnish

Directions: Heat the oil in a 3-quart saucepan. Add the onion, cover and cook gently for about 10 minutes or until beginning to brown, stirring frequently. Add garlic, turmeric, curry powder, ground cumin, and red pepper flakes, and cook, stirring, for 1 minute. Stir in the water, stock, lentils, barley, tomatoes, and salt and pepper to taste. Bring to a boil, cover and simmer about 45 minutes or until the lentils and barley are tender. Serve garnished with chopped fresh parsley or coriander. Nutrition: Serves 8. Per 1 cup serving: 180 calories, 12 grams protein, 5 grams fat, 25 grams carbohydrate.

HOT & SOUR SOUP: LACTO-OVO VEGETARIAN

This vegetarian soup provides ample protein with the inclusion of tofu. Be sure to stir fry the tofu cubes as directed for the best flavor.

2 medium red chilies, coarsely chopped
6 tablespoons rice vinegar
5 cups vegetable broth
2 stalks lemon grass, halved
4 tablespoons soy sauce, reduced sodium
1 tablespoon sugar
½ lime, juiced
2 tablespoons peanut oil
1 package (16 ounces) firm tofu, cubed
4 ounces mushrooms, sliced
4 medium scallions, chopped
1 cup bok choy (Chinese cabbage), shredded

Directions: Mix the chilies and vinegar together in a small non-reactive bowl. Cover and let stand at room temperature for 1 hour. Meanwhile, bring the vegetable broth to a boil in a 3-quart saucepan. Add the lemon grass, soy sauce, sugar, and lime juice, then reduce the heat and simmer for 20-30 minutes. Heat the oil in a preheated wok; add the tofu cubes and stir-fry over high heat for 2 to 3 minutes, or until browned all over. (You may need to do this in 2 batches, depending on the size of the wok.) Remove with a slotted spoon and drain on paper towels. Add the vinegar-chili mixture, mushrooms, tofu cubes, and half the scallions to the stock mixture and cook for 10 minutes. Mix the remaining scallions with the bok choy and use to garnish the soup before serving. Nutrition: Serves 6. Per 1-cup serving: 269 calories, 13 grams protein, 11 grams fat, 33 grams carbohydrate.

❋   *Soups and the Brown Bag Lunch*

It's a no-brainer that bringing lunch from home saves money and gives you total control over your nutrition. Soups make a great brown bag lunch. Remember to keep your food at the proper temperature including refrigeration until lunch break. Heat all leftovers to 180°F.

DAY 3: SOFT PROTEIN

Hump Day! How are you feeling?

As on Days 1 and 2, for the next three days you get to eat as much as you want as often as you want. But there is a catch: you must follow the plan. There are specific menu choices for Day 3. Today we introduce soft protein served in carefully measured portions. After two days of 5DPT liquids the introduction of soft protein is a welcome dietary change. It is likely on Day 3 you will start to feel that "newbie" tightness in your pouch. In addition, your hunger or carb cravings are likely to be diminished. Continue to observe the liquid restrictions and take your meals only on a "dry" pouch. Your dry pouch will hold soft protein longer prolonging feelings of satiety.

Protein Recommendations Day 3: canned fish (tuna or salmon) mixed with lemon and seasoned with salt and pepper, eggs cooked as desired seasoned with salt pepper and/or salsa, fresh soft fish (tilapia, sole, orange roughy), baked or grilled, and lightly seasoned. Yogurt and cottage cheese are allowed in ½-cup servings, and 1-ounce cheese servings, such as string cheese, are an acceptable between-meal snack provided liquid restrictions are followed. Vegetarian animal protein replacement products such as tofu or vegetable patties are acceptable on Day 3.

MOCHA PEANUT BUTTER BITES

✳   One of our most popular recipes!

Stir these together in a medium bowl and divide into 8 equal portions. Wrap each portion separately for a single serving. They are sure to cure your peanut butter blues.

1 (single serving) package instant high protein oatmeal
4 scoops chocolate protein powder
1 tablespoon flax seeds, ground
1/3 cup peanut butter, unsalted
¼ to ½-cup soymilk

Directions: With a spatula or wooden spoon blend all ingredients, adjusting the amount of soymilk to reach your desired consistency. Nutrition: Serves 8. Per serving: 141 calories, 14 grams protein, 6 grams fat, 8 grams carbohydrate.

✳   *Ingredient Note: Look for instant high protein oatmeal similar to Kashi® Go Lean Instant Oatmeal, available in most markets. If you prefer substitute reduced-fat evaporated milk for the soymilk.*

EGGS & BAKES

According to the American Egg Board, energy boosting foods are in demand. The humble chicken egg -nature's best answer in the quest for a near-perfect protein- can and should be a lead player in a diet high in protein. Consider the facts:

✳   Eggs contain the most easily digestible, most readily available protein compared to any other type.

✳   Eggs are used as the standard for measuring the protein quality of other ingredients.

✳   Processed eggs contribute the same high-quality protein as fresh.

These recipes take advantage of the protein value and nutritional benefits of eggs. In general, eggs are well-tolerated after gastric surgery and readily metabolized into energy and tissue building protein. Consider eggs for any meal of the day.

HARD-COOKED EGGS

As instructed by the American Egg Board: Place as many eggs as desired in a single layer in a saucepan. Add enough water to come at least 1 inch above the eggs. Cover saucepan and place on high heat and bring water to a boil. As soon as the water begins to boil turn off heat and remove saucepan from stove. Keep the saucepan covered and let eggs sit in the hot water for 12 to 15 minutes. When time is up run cold water over eggs to cool them. To remove shell, crackle it by tapping gently all over. Roll egg between hands to loosen shell. Peel the eggs starting at the large end. Hold egg under running cold water or dip in bowl of water to help ease off shell.

One egg provides 6 grams of protein, or 12% of the Recommended Daily Value (RDV) based on a 2000 calorie a day diet. Eggs provide the highest quality protein found in any food because they contain the essential amino acids our bodies need in a near-perfect pattern. While many people think the egg white has all the protein, the yolk actually provides nearly half of it.

The high-quality protein in eggs helps you to feel full longer and stay energized, which contributes to maintaining a healthy weight. In fact, research shows that eggs eaten at the start of the day can reduce daily calorie intake, prevent snacking between meals and keep you satisfied on those busy days when mealtime is delayed. Research indicates that high-quality protein may help active adults build muscle strength and middle-aged and aging adults prevent muscle loss. Consuming eggs following exercise is a great way to get the most benefits from exercise by encouraging muscle tissue repair and growth.

MOCK BREAKFAST BURRITO

Start your morning with this Mock Breakfast Burrito and you will have energy to burn. You may not be able to hold this full serving, so refrigerate leftovers for a snack if you get hungry later in the day

2 eggs or ½ cup egg substitute
cooking spray
1-ounce Cheddar cheese, shredded
2 tablespoons refried beans
1 tablespoon salsa

Directions: Measure the refried beans onto your plate and heat until warm in microwave. Set aside. Spray an 8-inch skillet with cooking spray and scramble eggs or egg substitute to desired doneness adding cheese in the last minute of cooking. Top heated beans with egg mixture and salsa. Nutrition: Serves 1. Per serving: 174 calories, 13 grams protein, 9 grams fat, 2 grams dietary fiber.

BREAKFAST BAKES

These hearty dishes are intended to energize your day from the very first bite. Breakfast bakes are high in protein, crazy good with flavor and easy to prepare and serve. Take the time to start your day with one of these dishes, which will satiate hunger and fuel your activities. Leftovers make great lunch selections to be quickly reheated in the workplace microwave oven.

✳ *Please Note: nutritional information is for a normal (FDA guidelines) serving size. It is expected that a weight loss surgery patient will eat only enough to fill their small stomach, which should be considerably less than a normal sized serving.*

BACON SWISS SQUARES

Traditional pork bacon infuses succulent flavor and richness to this breakfast bake. However, turkey bacon or vegetarian soy bacon may be substituted for the pork bacon with pleasing results.

2 cups biscuit baking mix (Bisquick®)
½ cup cold water
non-fat butter flavor cooking spray
8 ounces Swiss cheese, sliced
1-pound bacon, cooked and drained, chopped
4 whole eggs and 4 egg whites
(or substitute for the eggs an equivalent amount of pasteurized egg product such as egg beaters)
¼ cup milk

½ teaspoon onion powder

Directions: Heat the oven to 425°F. In a large bowl, combine the baking mix and water; stir 20 strokes. Turn onto a surface dusted with baking mix; knead 10 times. Spray a 13x9x2-inch glass baking dish with cooking spray. Press the dough into the bottom of the baking dish. Arrange cheese over dough. Sprinkle evenly with cooked chopped bacon. In a large bowl, whisk eggs, egg whites, milk and onion powder; pour over bacon. Bake on a lower rack in the heated oven for 15 to 18 minutes, or until a knife inserted near the center comes out clean. Cut into 12 equal pieces and serve immediately. Serves 12. Per serving: 372 calories, 18 grams protein, 27 grams fat, 14 grams carbohydrate.

✳ *Trouble Shooting: a soggy crust can be the result of high atmospheric humidity or higher moisture content in the eggs and other ingredients. To avoid soggy crust pre-bake the crust for 6 to 8 minutes in the heated oven before topping with cheese, bacon, and egg mixture. After topping the crust return the Bacon Swiss Squares to the oven and continue to bake 12-16 minutes until eggs are set and cooked through.*

SPINACH-SAUSAGE EGG BAKE

Spinach is a nutritional powerhouse loaded with beta carotene, folate, vitamin C, and the phytochemical lutein, which helps maintain vision. Surprisingly, spinach is also a good source of vegetable protein. Most WLS patients report good digestibility of spinach, specifically cooked spinach as in this recipe that uses frozen chopped spinach which has been thawed and squeezed dry.

1-pound country style sausage
1 small onion, chopped
cooking spray

1 (7-ounce) jar roasted red pepper, drained and chopped
1 (10-ounce) package chopped spinach, thawed, squeezed dry
1 cup all-purpose flour
¼ cup Parmesan cheese, grated
1 teaspoon dried basil
½ teaspoon salt
8 large eggs
2 cups milk, 2% low-fat
1 cup provolone cheese, shredded

Directions: Heat oven to 425°F. Coat a 3-quart baking dish with cooking spray, set aside. In a 10-inch skillet, cook sausage and onion over medium heat until meat is no longer pink; drain. Transfer to the prepared baking dish. Sprinkle with half of the red peppers; top with spinach. In a large bowl, combine the flour, Parmesan cheese, basil and salt. In another bowl whisk eggs and milk; stir into flour mixture until blended, but still lumpy. Pour over spinach. Bake, uncovered, for 15 to 20 minutes or until a knife inserted near the center comes out clean. Remove from oven, top with provolone cheese and remaining red peppers. Return to oven and bake 3 to 5 minutes or until cheese is melted. Let stand for 5 minutes before serving. Nutrition: Serves 6. Per serving: 638 calories, 30 grams protein, 45 grams fat, 27 grams carbohydrate. Very good served reheated for lunch the following day.

EGG BRUNCH BAKE

This recipe makes a generous casserole perfect for family brunch or potluck gatherings. It holds well on a buffet table and may be served at room temperature.

2 tablespoons butter
2 cups Cheddar cheese, shredded

2 cups cooked ham, cubed
12 large eggs
½ cup evaporated milk
2 teaspoons prepared mustard
salt and pepper, to taste

Directions: Drizzle butter into a 3-quart baking dish. Sprinkle with cheese and ham. In a mixing bowl, beat the eggs, evaporated milk, mustard, salt and pepper. Pour over ham and cheese. Bake uncovered, at 350°F for 40 to 45 minutes. Let stand for 5 to 10 minutes before serving. Nutrition: Serves 8. Per serving: 324 calories, 23 grams protein, 24 grams fat, 4 grams carbohydrate.

PUFFY TURKEY & SWISS OMELET

This quick omelet is a great breakfast, lunch, snack, or dinner for Day 3 of the pouch test. It is particularly appealing on Day 3 because the fluffy texture of the eggs is gentle on your freshly pampered pouch. I like to use the pre-cooked Jennie-O® Oven Roasted Premium Portion Turkey Breast.

butter-flavor cooking spray
¼ cup onion, finely chopped
½ cup cooked turkey breast, chopped
2 large egg whites (or equivalent egg white substitute)
¾ cup egg substitute
2 tablespoons water
salt and pepper to taste
1/3 cup Swiss cheese, reduced fat, shredded

Directions: Coat a 10-inch nonstick omelet pan or skillet with cooking spray; place over medium-high heat until hot. Add onion, cook and stir until tender. Add chopped turkey and cook and stir until warm. Slide to a small plate and tent with foil to keep warm. You will use this mixture to top the omelet in the final step.

In a medium bowl using an electric mixer beat egg whites at high speed until stiff peaks form (do not overbeat). In another large bowl whisk together the ¾-cup egg substitute, water, salt and pepper. Fold in the fluffy beaten egg white into egg substitute mixture.

Wipe the skillet clean with paper towels and coat with cooking spray. Place over medium heat until hot. Spread egg mixture in pan. Cover and reduce heat to low. Cook, covered for 5 minutes until puffy. Increase the heat to medium, uncover, and cook 3 minutes longer or until golden on bottom. Watch closely. Slide omelet to a serving plate, spread the turkey and onion mixture evenly on top and top with Swiss cheese. (If you like, slide the omelet under a preheated broiler to melt cheese). Slice into four equal portions. Serve warm. After the leftovers have cooled wrap in plastic or parchment paper and store refrigerated. Reheat gently in the microwave oven or enjoy at room temperature as a snack or meal. The leftover omelet is delicious with slices of fresh vine-ripe tomatoes. Nutrition: 4 Servings. Per serving: 88 calories, 12 grams protein, 3 grams fat, 3 grams carbohydrate.

TO-GO: CRANBERRY TURKEY ROLL-UPS

This is a terrific recipe to use on Day 3 and a great method to keep in mind when preparing portable meals to support your weight loss surgery diet. Experiment with different meats, cheese and condiments to add variety and interest to portable meals.

1-pound deli-style turkey, reduced sodium, sliced
4 ounces cream cheese spread with chives and onions
2 tablespoons cranberry sauce, no-sugar-added

Directions: Place two slices of turkey on a cutting board and spread with 1 teaspoon of cream cheese spread, and 1 teaspoon of cranberry sauce. Roll tightly, and secure with a toothpick and place in refrigerator container. Repeat with remaining ingredients and cover tightly with plastic wrap. Nutrition: Serves 4. Per serving: 232 calories, 27 grams protein, 10 grams fat, 5 grams carbohydrate.

FISH AND SEAFOOD SOFT PROTEIN

On Day 3 fish is the preferred menu option because it is soft and moist. In addition, fish canned in water is considered low fat and while we don't want to eliminate dietary fat reducing fat intake is prudent. However, for those with a fish allergy or fish aversion canned chicken or poultry may be substituted with similar results. For example, the Parmesan-Tuna Patties are a fan favorite. People abstaining from eating canned fish have enjoyed this recipe substituting canned chicken or canned turkey for the tuna.

PARMESAN TUNA PATTIES

＊ One of our most popular recipes!

By and far this is the favorite recipe of the 5 Day Pouch Test. In fact, after serving this recipe to the people at your table you can expect to have it requested by anyone with whom you share your lunch. Tuna is an outstanding source of lean protein at 27 grams per 4 ounce serving. Tuna provides plentiful amounts of healthful omega-3 fatty acids which contribute to healthy circulation and heart health.

Ingredients:

1 (6 ounce) can albacore tuna, in water

1 tablespoon mayonnaise

1 large egg

2 tablespoons Parmesan cheese

2 tablespoons ground flax meal

1 dash garlic powder

1 dash onion powder

1 dash salt

1 tablespoon olive oil or cooking spray

Directions: Drain tuna. Blend all ingredients in a medium size bowl and form into four equal patties. In a shallow skillet over medium high, heat the oil (I use olive oil, but cooking spray works equally well). Add tuna patties a cook until toasty brown, about three minutes, then turn and cook an additional 3 minutes. Serve warm or cold. Nutrition: Serves 4. Each tuna patty provides 132 calories, 16 grams protein, 7 grams fat, 2 grams carbohydrate.

✳ *Ingredient Note: Flax meal, made of ground flaxseed, is rich in omega-3 fatty acids which appear to help lower the risk of heart disease. Flaxseed adds a mild nutty flavor to foods and should be included regularly in a healthy diet. Weight loss surgery patients should use ground flax meal rather than flaxseed for ease of digestion.*

FISH CAKES

Fresh or frozen fish fillets are quickly poached and prepared with citrus to brighten the flavor. Thaw following package instructions.

1-pound firm fish fillets, cut into large chunks
½ teaspoon salt
¼ cup + 2 tablespoons 2% Greek yogurt
¼ cup chopped fresh parsley

1 egg yolk, beaten

1 tablespoon Dijon-style mustard

1 tablespoon freshly squeezed lemon juice (from 1/2 lemon)

¾ cup plus 2 tablespoons breadcrumbs

3 green onions, white parts minced

¼ teaspoon freshly ground black pepper

¼ cup canola oil

low-fat tartar sauce, optional

Directions: Steam fish: Put about an inch of water in bottom of large nonstick skillet and bring to a simmer over medium-high heat. Season fish with ¼ teaspoon of the salt and add it to the pan. Cover pan and simmer fish over low heat until just done, 6 to 8 minutes. Remove from pan with slotted spoon and drain on paper towels. Pour out the water and dry pan. Allow fish to cool slightly, about 5 minutes, and pat completely dry.

Flake fish in medium bowl with forks or your fingers, removing any bones as you go. Add yogurt, parsley, egg yolk, mustard, lemon juice, 6 tablespoons of the breadcrumbs, scallions, pepper, and remaining ¼-teaspoon salt. Stir to combine. Shape mixture into eight round cakes; coat cakes with remaining ½-cup breadcrumbs and shake off the excess.

Heat 2 tablespoons of the oil in the nonstick skillet over medium heat. Add fish cakes and cook until brown and crisp, 2 to 3 minutes. Add the remaining 2 tablespoons oil, turn cakes, and cook until golden brown on the other side, 2 to 3 minutes longer. Drain on paper towels. Serve hot with a low-fat tartar sauce, if desired. Nutrition: Serves 4; 2

fish patties per serving. Per serving: 291 calories, 29 grams protein, 14 grams fat, 12 grams carbohydrate.

SALMON PATTIES

Like other cold-water fish salmon is an excellent source of omega-3 fatty acids. In addition, canned salmon is a terrific source of. A 3-ounce serving of canned salmon provides 17 grams of protein along with vitamins B6 and B12 and niacin.

1 (14.75-ounce) can salmon with liquid, flaked
1 slice of bread, shredded
3 tablespoon chopped green onion, including the green parts
1 tablespoon fresh chopped dill weed, or 1 teaspoon dried
1 egg
½ teaspoon sweet paprika
salt and pepper to taste
1 tablespoon canola oil

Directions: In a large bowl, gently mix the salmon, bread, green onion, dill, egg, paprika, salt and pepper. Form into 8 patties; each about 1/2 inch thick. Heat oil over medium high heat in a 10-inch skillet. Cook the patties until nicely browned on both sides, about 3 to 4 minutes per side. Nutrition: Serves 4. Per serving (2 patties): 213 calories, 23 grams protein, 11 grams fat, 4 grams carbohydrate.

SALMON AND BLACK BEAN PATTIES

A high protein diet gets a boost of dietary fiber when beans are included in the meal. This salmon patty is fortified with canned black beans: a 1/3-cup serving provides a remarkable 10 grams dietary fiber. Black beans may be added whole or mashed as desired.

1 (7.5-ounce) can pink salmon, drained
½ cup canned black beans, rinsed and drained
¼ cup dry breadcrumbs
¼ cup sliced green onions
1 egg white
1 tablespoon lime juice
¼ teaspoon seafood seasoning
1 tablespoon canola oil

Directions: Place salmon in a medium bowl and break with fork. Add beans, breadcrumbs, green onions, egg white, lime juice and seasoning. Stir gently to combine. Shape mixture into four 1-inch thick patties. Refrigerate for 30 minutes or until ready to cook, no longer than 24 hours. Heat oil in a large skillet over medium heat: cook patties 2 to 3 minutes per side or until firm and brown. Season with salt and pepper and serve warm with tomato salsa. Nutrition: Serves two, 2 patties each. Per serving, 308 calories, 18 grams protein, 15 grams fat, 19 grams carbohydrate.

 ✳   *Shopping Hint: Select cod, halibut, tilapia or other firm textured white fish. Select a firm white fish that is free of bones and skins. Be sure to safely thaw frozen fish fillets following package instructions.*

QUICK LIST: DIETARY PROTEIN

Meat: beef, bison, lamb, game. The term meat is a broadly used term that includes beef, bison, lamb, and game meat. People following a high protein diet should select lean cuts of meat to reduce their intake of saturated fat.

Poultry. Chicken, turkey and other fowl are popular sources of lean protein for their ease in preparation and affordability. White meat poultry contains less fat than dark meat, but dark meat protein is a better source of vitamins and minerals.

Pork. Today's pork is leaner thanks to improved agriculture practices. Lean cuts include tenderloin, top loin, rib chops, and sirloin steak. Partake of cured pork products such as bacon, sausage, and ham in moderation.

Fish and shellfish. Perhaps the best source of lean protein combined with healthy fats, fish and shellfish support a well-planned high protein diet.

Beans and legumes. High protein diets tend to be low in dietary fiber. Including beans and legumes in meals provides the benefits of plant protein and dietary fiber in one healthy ingredient. A half cup serving of beans contains nearly the same protein as 3 ounces of broiled steak.

Low-fat dairy. Milk, cheese, and yogurt are not only protein-rich; they also provide calcium for strong bones and a healthy heart. Low-fat, or reduced fat dairy products provide the benefits of dairy with lowered calories.

DAY 3 NOTES:

DAY 4: FIRM PROTEIN

Look where you are: Day 4! Way to Go! You have the most difficult part of the 5 Day Pouch Test behind you and now is the time to start focusing on what you have learned and how you will use your new knowledge to eat and live well beyond the 5DPT.

Protein Recommendations: ground meat (beef, poultry, lamb, game) cooked dry and lightly seasoned; shellfish, scallops, lobster, steamed and seasoned with citrus, herbs and vegetables; salmon, or halibut steaks, grilled and lightly seasoned. Vegetarian products including tofu and vegetable burgers are acceptable.

Our Day 4 recipes feature firm protein fish, shellfish, seafood, ground poultry and meat prepared with fresh herbs, vegetables and fruit for your culinary enjoyment.

FISH AND SEAFOOD

Our global marketplace has made fish and seafood accessible and affordable. Salmon, tuna, and meaty fish such as swordfish, monkfish, and halibut are available fresh at most supermarkets. Along with plenty of high-quality protein, these lean satisfying fish supply B vitamins, potassium, and moderate amounts of omega-3 fatty acids. Consider including fish in your diet at least once a week to take advantage of the health supporting nutrients in your high protein diet. The fish and seafood recipes here are effective during the 5DPT on Day 4 and work well for your WLS and family menu beyond the Pouch Test.

HALIBUT WITH FETA-SPINACH TOPPING

The mild taste of halibut lends itself well to Greek seasoning and pungent feta cheese. Green spinach and red tomatoes make this dish visually appealing and rich in heart healthy phytochemicals. A small portion, served at room temperature, is a pleasing lunch. Other fish can be used for this recipe. At the market select seasonally fresh fish on the day it will be prepared.

4 (4-ounce) halibut fillets
2 teaspoons Greek seasoning, salt free
cooking spray
1 (10-ounce) package frozen chopped spinach, thawed and squeezed dry
1 plum tomato, coarsely chopped
¼ cup basil and tomato flavored feta cheese, crumbled

Directions: Season the halibut fillets evenly with the Greek seasoning. Coat a 10-inch skillet with cooking spray and heat over medium-high heat until hot. Add fish and cook 4 to 5 minutes, turn all fillets. Remove skillet from heat. Evenly divide the spinach, tomato and feta atop the fillets. Return skillet to heat, cover, and cook 4 minutes longer until spinach is hot, cheese has started to melt, and fish flakes easily when tested with a fork. Serve warm. Nutrition: Serves 4.

Per serving: 147 calories, 25 grams protein, 3 grams fat, 4 grams carbohydrate, 2 grams dietary fiber.

SUNFLOWER ORANGE ROUGHY

Orange roughy, sometimes called sea perch, is a relatively large deep-sea fish with a firm flesh of mild flavor. It is sold skinned and filleted, fresh or frozen. This crispy crust and tender meat preparation is flavorful and satisfying while being protein dense. The inclusion of corn flake crumbs adds crunch without turning this into a starchy carbohydrate-heavy recipe. Other soft fish may be used in place of the orange roughy. This is a good reheated lunch on Day 5.

¼ cup corn flake crumbs
2 tablespoons dry roasted sunflower kernels
1 teaspoon salt-free all-purpose seasoning blend
4 (4-ounce) orange roughy fillets
1 tablespoon lemon juice
cooking spray

Directions: Heat oven to 425°F. On a piece of waxed paper combine the corn flake crumbs, sunflower kernels, and seasoning blend. Place orange roughy fillets on a plate and sprinkle with lemon juice. Dip fillets in corn flake mixture and press crumbs to adhere to fish. Place on a foil-lined baking sheet lightly sprayed with cooking spray. Use any remaining crumb mixture to press on fish. Bake the fish on the middle rack in a heated oven for 10 to 12 minutes or until fish is done. Serve warm. Nutrition: Serves 4. Per serving: 201 calories, 23 grams protein, 9 grams fat, 6 grams carbohydrate. Ingredient Note: Sunflower seeds are packed with vitamin E and folate. They also provide reasonable amounts of magnesium, copper, iron, and zinc.

SALMON WITH MUSTARD CREAM SAUCE

Salmon is rich in omega-3 fatty acids which appear to have several health benefits including lowering triglycerides, maintaining heart rhythm, and decreasing the risk of clot formation in the arteries. Once you have completed the 5DPT consider including salmon in your menu at least once a week to take advantage of its health promoting nutrients.

4 (4 to 6-ounce) skinless salmon fillets
cooking spray
black pepper
½ cup sour cream, reduced fat
1½ tablespoons Dijon-style mustard
2 teaspoons fresh dill, chopped
1½ teaspoons lemon juice
1 clove garlic, minced
¼ teaspoon salt

Directions: Preheat broiler and spray broiler pan lightly with cooking spray. Place salmon fillets on a broiler pan, and spray them lightly with cooking spray, season with black pepper. Broil 8 to 10 minutes or until salmon flakes when tested with a fork. Sauce: Meanwhile, in a small bowl combine sour cream, Dijon-style mustard, fresh dill, ¼ teaspoon black pepper, lemon juice, garlic, and salt. Place one filet on each plate and garnish with 2 tablespoons of the Mustard Cream Sauce. Serve warm, 1 fillet per person, with 2 tablespoons of sauce. Nutrition: Serves 4 (1 fillet and 2 tablespoons sauce). Per serving: 254 calories, 36 grams protein, 10 grams fat, 3 grams carbohydrate.

ORANGE GLAZED SALMON

This succulent salmon includes freshly squeezed orange juice and fresh orange slices.When we include a sweet taste with a firm protein, such as this fresh citrusy-orange glaze with salmon, after dinner sweet cravings are diminished.

4 (4 to 6-ounce) salmon fillets
salt and pepper to taste
cooking spray
3 tablespoons soy sauce, reduced sodium
1 orange, zest grated and reserved, juiced
2 oranges, sliced

Directions: Season salmon fillets to taste with salt and pepper. Coat a 10-inch skillet with cooking spray, heat over medium-high. Add salmon and cook 4 to 6 minutes per side until fish is done. Remove to a plate and tent loosely with foil. Return skillet to pan, add orange juice, orange zest, and soy sauce. Increase heat to high and stir and cook for 1-minute to deglaze the pan and slightly reduce the sauce. Place each salmon fillet on a plate, top with 1 tablespoon of sauce and serve warm with orange slices. Nutrition: Serves 4. Per serving: 148 calories, 23 grams protein, 4 grams fat, 1 gram carbohydrate.

✳ *Recipe Note: If you plan to use the leftovers for a future meal, refrigerate the cooked salmon and the sauce separately. Reheat leftovers gently in the microwave to avoid over cooking.*

TUNA STEAKS WITH SALSA & AVOCADO

Healthy Avocado: The fat content is higher in this recipe because of the 5 grams of monounsaturated from the avocado.

Monounsaturated fats are known to help reduce the levels of LDL (the bad) cholesterol. In addition, the richness of the avocado is particularly satiating, and tends to reduce post-meal hunger cravings.

> 4 (4 to 6-ounce) tuna steaks
> Mrs. Dash® Garlic & Herb Seasoning Blend, to taste
> 1 tablespoon olive oil
> 1 cup salsa
> 1 avocado cut in 8 slices

Directions: Season tuna steaks to taste with the garlic and herb seasoning blend. In a 10-inch skillet heat the olive oil over medium-high heat until hot. Add tuna steaks and cook 3 to 4 minutes on each side until done. Meanwhile, warm the salsa in the microwave oven. Serve each tuna steak topped with ¼ cup of salsa and two slices avocado. Nutrition: Serves 4. Per serving: 188 calories, 27 grams protein, 13 grams fat, 6 grams carbohydrate.

✳ *Method Note: the tuna steaks may also be cooked on an outdoor gas or charcoal grill over medium-high direct heat.*

SESAME TUNA

Sesame seed has a nutty, slightly sweet flavor that makes it versatile enough for use in baked goods such as breads, pastries, cakes, and cookies as well as an interesting ingredient for savory dishes. History tells us this is the earliest known seasoning. The addition of sesame seeds to protein creates a nutty flavor and texture improving the enjoyment of the meal. Find sesame seeds in the spice aisle. Sesame seeds turn rancid quickly because of their natural oils: pay close attention to the expiration date and smell or taste for freshness before adding to a recipe and potentially spoiling all ingredients.

½ teaspoon salt
4 (4 to 6-ounce) tuna steaks
2 tablespoons sesame seeds
2 teaspoons sesame oil
12 green onion tops, cut into 2-inch strips
1 tablespoon soy sauce, reduced sodium

Directions: Season tuna steaks with salt, and then sprinkle sesame seeds on both sides of each steak pressing gently into fish. Heat the sesame oil in a 12-inch skillet over medium-high heat. Add tuna and cook for 2 to 4 minutes on each side or until fish flakes easily when tested with a fork. Remove from pan to serving platter, and tent loosely with foil to keep warm. Add green onions and soy sauce to pan and cook and stir for 3 minutes until green onions are tender. Divide evenly over tuna fillets. Serve warm, 1 fillet per serving. Nutrition: Serves 4. Per serving: 249 calories, 41 grams protein, 6 grams fat, 5 grams carbohydrate.

PARMESAN BAKED FISH

This mayonnaise-Parmesan topping is great on baked firm-flesh fish of all kinds. Use frozen fish fillets that have been thawed per package directions or select the freshest fillet from your fish market on the day the recipe will be prepared. This is a fantastic dish and method to include on your Day 6 and beyond menu.

¼ cup low-fat mayonnaise or salad dressing
2 tablespoons grated Parmesan cheese
1 tablespoon snipped fresh chives or sliced green onion

1 teaspoon Worcestershire sauce
cooking spray
4 (4 to 6-ounce) fresh or frozen and thawed skinless fish fillets

Directions: Sauce. In a small bowl stir together mayonnaise, Parmesan cheese, chives, and Worcestershire sauce. Set aside. Baked Fish. Heat oven to 450°F degrees. Rinse fish; pat dry with paper towels. Place fish in a 2-quart square or rectangular baking dish coated with cooking spray. Spread mayonnaise mixture evenly over fish. Bake, uncovered, in heated oven for 12 to 15 minutes, or until fish flakes easily when tested with a fork. Nutrition: 145 calories, 21 grams protein, 6 grams fat, 1 gram carbohydrate. Nutrition based on average cold-water fish; refer to package labeling for nutritional data specific to your ingredients.

BUTTERY LEMON SHRIMP

This is a healthy take on the classic shrimp scampi. Reheat leftovers gently for an enjoyable afternoon snack or toss with scrambled eggs for a protein dense breakfast on Days 4 and 5 and Beyond the 5DPT.

zest of 1 lemon
1 tablespoon fresh chives, chopped
¼ cup yogurt-based spread (see note)
2 tablespoons lemon juice
1 teaspoon Worcestershire sauce
½ teaspoon paprika
1 tablespoon olive oil
1 pound peeled and deveined large shrimp
1 teaspoon Old Bay® Seafood Seasoning

Directions: Combine lemon zest with chopped chives and set aside. In a small bowl mix the yogurt-based spread, lemon juice, Worcestershire sauce, and paprika. Set aside. Place the olive oil in a 10-inch skillet over medium heat. Add the shrimp and Old Bay® Seafood Seasoning and cook and stir until shrimp turns pink. Add the yogurt spread and continue cooking until shrimp are done. Divide shrimp and sauce evenly among four bowls and garnish with the lemon zest and chives. Nutrition: Serves 4. Per serving: 171 calories, 26 grams protein, 6 grams fat, trace of carbohydrate. Ingredient

✳   *Ingredient Note: At our home we love the healthy and yogurt-based spread Brummel & Brown. It is heat stable and has a creamy buttery taste. Brummel & Brown is 35% vegetable oil and 10% non-fat yogurt. It is made in the USA by Unilever.*

SPICY STIR-FRY SHRIMP

This is a quick and easy recipe that can be adapted for Day 6 and beyond by adding your favorite blend of stir-fry vegetables to the bell pepper, celery, and green onions.

1 tablespoon canola oil
1 red bell pepper, sliced into thin strips
1 rib celery, sliced diagonally into ½ inch pieces
4 green onions, sliced diagonally into ½ inch pieces
1 teaspoon Mrs. Dash® Extra Spicy Seasoning Blend
1/3 cup chicken broth, reduced sodium
1-pound large shrimp, peeled and deveined

Directions: In a large (12-inch) skillet or wok heat the canola oil to very hot. Add bell pepper strips, celery slices, and green onions. Cook and stir until vegetables are just tender. Add spicy seasoning blend and chicken broth, stir to combine. Add the shrimp, continue stirring and cooking over high heat until shrimp turn pink and are opaque in the center. Adjust seasoning to taste with the spice blend, salt and pepper. Serve warm. Nutrition: Serves 4. Per serving: 178 calories, 29 grams protein, 5 grams fat, 4 grams carbohydrate.

CITRUS BAY SCALLOPS

Bay scallops are generally harvested only on the East Coast but are widely available in the United States, fresh and frozen. They are small: the muscle is about ½-inch in diameter. The meat of the bay scallop is sweeter and more succulent than that of the larger sea scallop. They cook quickly; watch closely to avoid over-cooking.

1 tablespoon olive oil
1-pound bay scallops
2 tablespoons lemon juice
1 tablespoon chopped fresh parsley, plus sprigs for garnish
1 teaspoon grated orange zest
2 cloves garlic, minced (optional)
salt and pepper to taste

Directions: In a 10-inch skillet set on medium-high, heat the olive oil. While it heats in a medium bowl toss together the bay scallops, lemon juice, chopped parsley, orange zest, and minced garlic. When oil is hot add scallop mixture and cook and stir until scallops are done. Season with salt and pepper to taste, and garnish with parsley sprigs. Serve warm. Nutrition: Serves 4. Per serving: 185 calories, 29 grams protein, 5 grams fat, 5 grams carbohydrate.

✳ *Recipe Note: Serve the leftovers, chilled, over mixed greens with light citrus vinaigrette. This makes a healthy, portable, and mouthwatering Day 6 lunch.*

PAN-SEARED SCALLOPS WITH CHERRY TOMATOES

Sea scallops are about 1½ inches in diameter. The meat is chewy, sweet, and moist. They must be cooked quickly to avoid becoming rubbery. In addition to pan searing they are used in soups, stews, and salads. This recipe requires quick cooking over very high heat. A 3-ounce serving of sea scallops is only 75 calories and contains 14 grams protein with only trace amounts of fat and carbohydrate.

1-pound sea scallops, fresh (or frozen and thawed)
1 tablespoon olive oil
1 (8-ounce) package cherry tomatoes
2 tablespoons balsamic vinegar
2 tablespoons fresh basil, chopped

Directions: Heat the olive oil in a 10-inch heavy-bottom skillet over high heat. When the oil is hot add the scallops and allow them to sear and cook quickly, do not disturb or the flesh will tear. As the scallops become opaque, carefully turn and cook another 2 to 3 minutes until done. Remove to a plate and tent loosely with foil to keep warm. Lower heat to medium-high. Add cherry tomatoes to skillet. Cook and stir until tomato skins just begin to pop. Stir in balsamic vinegar and fresh basil, and cook another minute, stirring to coat all tomatoes. Serve warm tomatoes, with scallops, drizzling with the balsamic vinegar pan sauce. Nutrition: Serves 4. Per serving: 123 calories, 20 grams protein, 1 gram fat, 7 grams carbohydrate.

GROUND MEAT AND POULTRY

Ground meat and poultry are affordable and readily available in most markets. Many weight loss surgery patients who include lean ground meat and poultry in their diet report good digestibility and satiation. In addition, meals made with ground meat and poultry can be shared among family and friends without complaints about diet food. Try these recipes and enjoy the menu on Day 4 of the 5 Day Pouch Test and countless healthy meals for Day 6 and beyond.

SLOW COOKER THAI PEANUT MEATBALLS

This convenient slow cooker recipe cooks in just 2 hours on high heat. With only three convenient ingredients it makes the grade for a terrific weeknight family friendly meal. For Day 4 enjoy 2 to 4 meatballs: stop eating at the first sign of fullness. For the family and meals beyond the 5DPT serve the meatballs with rice and stir-fried vegetables for a balanced meal.

> 1 (13.5-ounce) can coconut milk
> 1 (3.5-ounce) box A Taste of Thai® Peanut Sauce Mix
> 1 (16-ounce) package frozen beef meatballs
> sliced green onion and lime wedges for garnish

Directions: In the bowl of the crockpot whisk together the coconut milk and peanut sauce mix. Add the frozen meatballs and stir until all meatballs are coated with the sauce. Cover and cook on high for 2 hours, stirring once during cooking. Serve warm drizzled with sauce. Nutrition: Serves 4. Four meatballs per serving: 350 calories, 18 grams protein, 22 grams fat, 14 grams carbohydrate.

TURKEY-PARMESAN-PESTO MEATBALLS

These meatballs come together quickly and have a rich flavor from the pesto sauce. The onion helps keep the lean meat moist. They are good broken and included in scrambled eggs for breakfast on Day

5. Pesto is an uncooked sauce made with fresh basil, garlic, pine nuts, parmesan or Pecorino cheese and olive oil. The ingredients can either be crushed with mortar and pestle or finely chopped with a food processor. This classic, fresh-tasting sauce originated in Genoa, Italy. There are many finely crafted artisanal pesto sauces available today at supermarkets and farmer's markets.

1½ pounds ground turkey, white meat only
¼ cup pesto sauce
1/3 cup Parmesan cheese, grated
1 small white onion, finely chopped
½ teaspoon salt
additional pesto for dipping

Directions: Heat oven to 375°F. In large bowl, gently combine ground turkey, ¼-cup pesto, Parmesan cheese, onion and salt. Shape mixture into 30 equal meatballs. Place meatballs on a wire rack above a foil-lined rimmed baking sheet. Make sure they are not touching. Bake in the heated oven for 15 to 20 minutes. Serve warm with additional pesto sauce for dipping. Nutrition: Serves 6. Per (4-meatball) serving: 202 calories, 31 grams protein, 7 grams fat, 2 grams carbohydrate.

VEGGIE MUSHROOM-SWISS PATTY MELTS

For vegetarians who eat dairy products (*lacto ovo vegetarians*) this is a delicious and satiating Day 4 recipe that can be made ahead and reheated in the microwave for an easy meal. Consider Veggie Mushroom-Swiss Patty Melts for your portable Day 5 lunch.

4 (2.8 ounce) frozen vegetarian burger (such as Boca Burger®)
¼ cup chicken stock, reduced sodium

1 (8 ounce) package sliced mushrooms
1 small onion, chopped
black pepper, to taste
cooking spray
4 (1 ounce) slices Swiss cheese, reduced fat

Directions: Preheat oven broiler. In a 10-inch skillet cook veggie burgers according to package directions. Set aside and keep warm. In the same cooking pan heat the chicken stock, scraping any browned bits from the pan. Add the mushrooms, and onion, and cook and stir over medium-high heat until the vegetables are tender. On a foil lined cookie sheet prayed with cooking spray place the four veggie patties and divide the mushroom mixture evenly on top of each burger. Place one slice of Swiss cheese on each burger. Place under broiler to melt cheese. Watch closely to avoid burning. Serve warm. Nutrition: Serves 4. Per serving: 162 calories, 23 grams protein, 5 grams fat, 9 grams carbohydrate.

✳ *Recipe Note: You may also use this recipe preparation using an equal portion ground meat or poultry patty.*

CLASSIC SALISBURY STEAK

Classic comfort food, Salisbury steak is traditionally a ground beef patty flavored with minced onion and seasonings before being fried or broiled. It was named after a 19th-century English physician, Dr. J. H. Salisbury, who recommended that his patients eat plenty of beef for all manner of ailments. Salisbury steak is often served with gravy made from pan drippings. To suit our different tastes this recipe may be prepared with ground beef, pork or white meat poultry.

1-pound ground meat of your choice

1/3 cup dry breadcrumbs

½ teaspoon salt

¼ teaspoon pepper

1 egg

1 large onion, sliced

1 can (14.5 ounces) condensed beef broth

1 can (4 ounces) sliced mushrooms, drained

cooking spray

2 tablespoons cold water

2 teaspoons cornstarch

Directions: Mix ground meat, breadcrumbs, salt, pepper and egg: shape into four equal size patties. Over medium-high heat, cook patties in 10-inch skillet sprayed with cooking spray. Turn patties occasionally cooking until brown, about 10 to 12 minutes. Remove to a plate and tent loosely with foil to keep warm. Drain excess fat from skillet. Add onion, broth, and mushrooms, cook and stir to bring browned bits up from pan. In a small bowl whisk together water and cornstarch, then whisk cornstarch mixture into onion mixture, still cooking over medium-high heat. Return patties to pan and simmer about 10 minutes until sauce reduces, and meat patties are cooked and tender. Serve meat patties with ¼ cup of sauce per serving.

Nutrition Note: Below nutrition data is provided for ground beef, pork, and white meat poultry: 1 meat patty with ¼ cup sauce.

Per serving using extra lean ground beef: 321 calories, 27 grams protein, 21 grams fat, 6 grams carbohydrate and 1 gram dietary fiber.

Per serving using lean ground pork: 354 calories, 24 grams protein, 25 grams fat, 6 grams carbohydrate and 1 gram dietary fiber.

Per serving using ground white meat poultry: 225 calories, 25 grams protein, 11 grams fat, 6 grams carbohydrate and 1 gram dietary fiber.

WHAT IF CARB CRAVINGS COME BACK AFTER THE 5DPT?

Go Green! Including vegetables in our weight loss surgery diet is not only smart nutrition; it honestly helps tame carbohydrate cravings. Vegetables are complex carbohydrates. They deliver nutrients, minerals, and vitamins to our body and affect blood glucose levels naturally. They give us color and crunch and are willing participants in any preparation from raw and dipped to oven roasted and seasoned with herbs and spices. Remember to follow the 2B/1B rhythm: 2 Bites Protein to 1 Bite Carbohydrate (including vegetable carbohydrate) to keep Protein First in your meal plan. Here are some tips from the USDA for preparing vegetables and enjoying them as part of your healthy plate:

* Buy fresh vegetables in season. They cost less and are likely to be at their peak flavor.

* Stock up on frozen vegetables for quick and easy cooking in the microwave.

* Buy vegetables that are easy to prepare. Pick up pre-washed bags of salad greens and add baby carrots or grape tomatoes for a salad in minutes. Buy packages of veggies such as baby carrots or celery sticks for quick snacks.

* Use a microwave to quickly "zap" vegetables. White or sweet potatoes can be baked quickly this way.

* Vary your veggie choices to keep meals interesting.

* Think soup. Our carb monster soups are perfect year-round for taming the carb-hungry beast within us all.

DAY 5: SOLID PROTEIN

Day 5 and you did it! I knew you could. This is your final day of the 5DPT and your re-entry into the healthy way of eating that will allow you to lose or maintain weight, manage your blood sugar, and simply feel good: isn't that the ultimate goal? Protein choices include poultry, beef, pork and anything from Day 4. Here are several dinner recipes you can enjoy on Day 5 and beyond. Bring forward some breakfast ideas from Day 3 and lunch ideas from Day 4 for a full day of chewing, eating, satiety, and loving that sweet little working pouch of yours.

CHICKEN AND POULTRY

CHIPOTLE-JALAPENO CHICKEN WITH BLACK BEANS

This flavorful chicken and bean recipe is a quick easy weeknight meal on Day 5. The added fiber from the beans is filling and nutritious.

1 tablespoon Mrs. Dash® Southwest Chipotle Seasoning Blend
4 (4-ounce) chicken breasts halves, skinless, boneless
cooking spray
½ cup Monterey Jack cheese with jalapeno peppers, shredded

79

2 tablespoons canned jalapeno peppers, diced
1 (15-ounce) can black beans, rinsed and drained
¼ cup mild salsa

Directions: Season both sides of the chicken pieces with the Southwest Chipotle Seasoning. Coat a 12-inch skillet with cooking spray and place over high heat. When heated add chicken to pan and cook 7 to 10 minutes on each side until done. While the chicken cooks, put beans and salsa in a medium sized microwave safe bowl and heat on high power 3 to 4 minutes, until warm, stirring once. Remove chicken from heat; sprinkle with cheese. Cover to allow cheese to melt and serve garnished with sliced jalapenos. Nutrition: Serves 4. Per serving: 282 calories, 35 grams protein, 8 grams fat, 15 grams carbohydrate, and 6 grams dietary fiber.

MUSTARD BAKED CHICKEN

This is an easy baked dish that is good for cooler evenings. If you prefer to use ready-to-cook boneless skinless chicken pieces in place of the bone-in fryer chicken pieces. It may also be prepared in a slow cooker using frozen chicken pieces and cooking on high 2 to 4-hours or low 4 to 6-hours.

1 (2½ to 3½ lbs.) broiler-fryer chicken, cut up
cooking spray
1/3 cup brown mustard
1 tablespoon cooking oil
1 tablespoon soy sauce, reduced sodium
2 teaspoons heat-stable granular sugar substitute

Directions: Heat oven to 425°F. If desired, remove skin from chicken. Place chicken in a 3-quart rectangular baking dish coated with cooking spray. Bake in a preheated oven for 15 minutes.

Meanwhile, in a small bowl stir together mustard, oil, soy sauce, and sugar substitute. Remove chicken from oven. Generously brush mustard mixture over chicken. Return to oven and continue baking for 25 minutes or until chicken is tender and no longer pink. Baste occasionally with mustard mixture. Serve warm topped with sauce from baking dish. Nutrition: Serves 6. Per serving: 259 calories, 14 grams 4 grams carbohydrate and 29 grams protein.

PEPPER-LIME CHICKEN

This chicken cooks quickly under the broiler and brings a Caribbean flair to the table. Try boneless, skinless chicken thighs if you prefer dark meat chicken.

6 (4-ounce) chicken breast halves or thighs, boneless, skinless
1 teaspoon finely shredded lime peel
¼ cup lime juice
1 tablespoon canola oil
1 teaspoon dried thyme, crushed
1 teaspoon bottled minced garlic
salt and pepper to taste

Directions: Preheat broiler. Place chicken on the unheated rack of a broiler pan. Broil 4 to 5-inches from the heat for 10 minutes or until chicken starts to brown. Meanwhile, for glaze, in a small bowl stir together lime peel, lime juice, canola oil, thyme, garlic, salt, and pepper. Brush chicken with glaze. Turn chicken; brush with more glaze. Broil for 5 to 15 minutes more or until chicken is tender and no longer pink, brushing with the remaining glaze the final 5 minutes of broiling. Nutrition: Serves 6. Per serving: 242 calories, 28 grams protein, 13 grams fat, 2 grams carbohydrate

CHICKEN WITH CANNELLINI BEANS

Lean chicken with fiber-dense beans is a healthy and satisfying Day 5 meal that can be enjoyed in your ongoing pursuit of health after the 5 Day Pouch Test. The sun-dried tomato sprinkles can be found in the produce section of your supermarket.

cooking spray
4 (4-ounce) boneless skinless chicken breast halves
1 teaspoon dried rosemary
salt and pepper to taste
1 cup chicken broth, fat-free, **reduced sodium**
1 (16-ounce) can cannellini beans, drained and rinsed
2 tablespoons sun-dried tomato sprinkles

Directions: Coat a 12-inch skillet with cooking spray and heat over medium heat until hot. Add chicken, and season with rosemary, salt, and pepper. Cook 6 to 8 minutes and turn, add chicken broth, cannellini beans, and sun-dried tomato sprinkles to skillet. Bring to a brisk simmer, reduce heat, cover and cook additional 6 minutes or more until done. Serve chicken and cannellini beans warm, drizzled with sauce. Nutrition: Serves 4. Per serving: 193 calories, 30 grams protein, 2 grams fat, 11 grams carbohydrate, 4 grams dietary fiber.

SLOW COOKER CHICKEN PARMESAN

Everyone loves chicken Parmesan and this one will be ready when you get home from work. Cook spinach fettuccine for the family but enjoy yours without it. This makes great lunch leftovers for Day 6 and beyond.

3 pounds chicken pieces, boneless and skinless
1 (14.5-ounce) can Italian style tomatoes

1 (6-ounce) can tomato paste
1 small onion, chopped
1 teaspoon dried Mrs. Dash® Italian Seasoning Blend
½ cup Parmesan cheese, grated

Directions: Place frozen chicken pieces in a 4-quart slow cooker. In a small bowl combine tomatoes, tomato paste, onion and Italian seasoning blend, and pour over chicken pieces. Cover and set at high for 2 to 4-hours or low for 4 to 6-hours. Serve warm with sauce sprinkled with Parmesan cheese. Serving is 4-ounces chicken and 1/3 cup sauce and 1 tablespoon Parmesan cheese. Nutrition: Per serving: 202 calories, 28 grams protein, 5 grams fat, 10 grams carbohydrate.

CHICKEN AND EDIBLE POD PEAS

The fresh crunch of quick-cooked pea pods and the refreshing lemon-pepper seasoning make this a light and healthy lunch or dinner on Day 5 and beyond. Edible pod peas are sometimes called snap peas, sugar-snap peas, or snow peas.

cooking spray, butter flavor
2 teaspoons lemon-pepper seasoning
4 (4-ounce) chicken breasts, boneless and skinless
¼ cup yogurt-based spread
1 (6-ounce) package sugar snap peas

Directions: Spray a 10-inch skillet with cooking spray and heat over medium-high heat. Season the chicken breasts with the lemon-pepper seasoning, and cook in the skillet, 8 to 12 minutes turning occasionally. Remove to a serving plate and tent loosely with foil to keep warm. Return skillet to heat and add yogurt-based spread and sugar snap peas. Cook and stir for 4 to 5 minutes until just tender. Serve with warm chicken, spooning sauce over peas and chicken.

83

Nutrition: Serves 4. Per serving: 259 calories, 35 grams protein, 8 grams fat, 5 grams carbohydrate.

SLOW COOKER GARLIC & THYME CHICKEN THIGHS

Take the guesswork out of Day 5 dinner when you throw this in the slow cooker first thing in the morning. The sweet orange and balsamic sauce makes everyday chicken into a gourmet's delight.

6 (4-ounce) frozen boneless, skinless chicken thighs
1-2 tablespoons bottled minced garlic
1½ teaspoons dried thyme
salt and pepper to taste
½ cup orange juice
2 tablespoons balsamic vinegar
2 oranges, sliced

Directions: Place frozen chicken thighs in a 3½ to 4-quart slow cooker. In a small bowl whisk together the garlic, thyme, salt, pepper, orange juice, and balsamic vinegar and pour over chicken thighs. Cover and set to low-heat for 6 to 8-hours or high-heat for 2 to 4-hours. Just before serving strain juices into a 1-quart saucepan and bring to a boil to reduce liquid. Boil gently, uncovered, for about 10 minutes or until reduced to about 1 cup. Serve 1 thigh topped with 1 tablespoon sauce and orange slices. Nutrition: Serves 6. Per serving: 178 calories, 34 grams protein, 4 grams fat, 5 grams carbohydrate.

TURKEY-AVOCADO-SWISS STACK

This is a take on a sandwich served at one of my favorite restaurants. The restaurant serves it on toasted marble rye bread. I have adapted it at home to simply be a high protein stack served on a plate, eaten with a fork.

16 ounces oven roasted turkey breast, sliced
4 teaspoons Miracle Whip® light
1 large avocado, sliced
4 (1-ounce) slices reduced-fat Swiss cheese
2 ounces sprouts
salt and pepper to taste

Directions: On each of four salad plates arrange 4-ounces of turkey breast slices. Spread each stack with 1 teaspoon of Miracle Whip® light. Arrange the avocado slices, sprouts, and Swiss cheese on top of each stack. Season with salt and pepper. Serve chilled. Nutrition: Serves 4. Per serving: 275 calories, 35 grams protein, 12 grams fat, 6 grams carbohydrate.

TURKEY TENDERLOIN WITH MUSTARD MUSHROOM SAUCE

The mustard mushroom sauce is rich and creamy which contributes to feelings of fullness and satiation. This is a company-worthy main dish.

1½ tablespoons Mrs. Dash® Original Seasoning Blend
2 tablespoons flour
1-pound turkey tenderloin, cut into 1-inch cutlets
2 teaspoons olive oil
1 (8-ounce) package sliced mushrooms
3/4 cup chicken broth, reduced sodium
1½ tablespoons coarse-grain mustard
2 tablespoons heavy cream

Directions: In a medium bowl combine 1 tablespoon of seasoning blend with the flour. Dredge the turkey cutlets with the flour mixture. Heat the olive oil in a 10-inch skillet over medium-high heat, add the turkey cutlets and cook until golden brown on both sides. Remove turkey from skillet to a rimmed plate and tent with foil to keep warm. Return skillet to heat and add sliced mushrooms. Stir and cook until the mushrooms are tender. Pour chicken broth over mushrooms and cook, scraping brown pieces from bottom of the pan. Add the mustard and ½ tablespoon of seasoning blend to the sauce and mix well. Add the heavy cream and cook and stir until the sauce is thick and well combined. Return turkey cutlets to pan with sauce to reheat. Serve each cutlet drizzled with sauce. Nutrition: Serves 4. Per serving: 272 calories, 28 grams protein, 14 grams fat, 7 grams carbohydrate.

PORK: THE OTHER WHITE MEAT

Pork is fast becoming a weight-conscious persons favorite white meat thanks, in part, to a 2011 Purdue University study that concluded including protein from lean pork in the diet promotes weight loss and preserves lean muscle mass for those who are dieting. Additionally, dieters eating pork rated themselves more positively in terms of mood and feelings of pleasure compared to a menu void of pork.

The USDA and National Pork Board recommend using a digital instant-read thermometer to ensure pork is cooked to 145ºF for a moist succulent piece of lean pork.

Today's pork is lean and nutrient rich and a very good source of protein. If you cannot find boneless pork tenderloin chops purchase vacuum sealed pork tenderloin and slice into 1-inch thick chops.

SEARED PORK TENDERLOIN CHOPS WITH BALSAMIC SAUCE
½ cup balsamic vinegar
½ cup beef broth, **reduced sodium**
4 (4-ounce) pork tenderloin chops, boneless and trimmed of fat

salt and pepper to taste

1 tablespoon olive oil

Directions: Make sauce. Place balsamic vinegar and beef broth in a 1-quart saucepan and heat to a simmer over medium-high. Simmer until sauce is reduced and thickened, about 6 to 8 minutes. For Chops: season chops with salt and pepper on both sides. On stovetop, heat oil in a 10-inch skillet over medium-high heat. When oil is hot cook chops 5 to 8 minutes on each side, turning only once. Internal temperature should be 145°F. Serve each chop with 1 tablespoon of the balsamic sauce. Nutrition: Serves 4. Per serving: 213 calories, 25 grams protein, 10 grams fat, 5 grams carbohydrate.

SKILLET PORK CHOPS WITH HONEY-MUSTARD SAUCE

The pork here is served with spinach, which adds fiber and nutrients to the meal, yet it remains low in carbohydrates and high in protein. Using pre-marinated pork tenderloin makes preparation swift and takes the guesswork out of seasoning.

1 (24-ounce) honey-mustard marinated pork tenderloin

pepper to taste

cooking spray

3 tablespoons lemon juice

4 green onions, finely chopped

1 (16-ounce) package frozen spinach, thawed and squeezed dry

Directions: Cut the tenderloin into six equal slices and season each slice with pepper to taste. Heat a 12-inch skillet sprayed with cooking spray over medium-high heat until hot. Add pork and cook, 4 to 6 minutes per side or until done. Remove pork to a rimmed plate and tent loosely with foil. Add lemon juice and green onions to skillet and cook and stir until onions are tender. Stir in spinach, and cook, stirring constantly for 2 to 3 minutes. Divide spinach mixture among six serving plates and top each with 1 slice of pork tenderloin. Nutrition: Serves 6. Per serving: 166 calories, 23 grams protein, 5 grams fat, 5 grams carbohydrate.

BEEF & OTHER RED MEAT

Meat: beef, bison, lamb, game. The term meat is a broadly used term that includes beef, bison, lamb, and game meat. People following a high protein diet should select lean cuts of meat to reduce their intake of saturated fat.

SIRLOIN STEAKS WITH HORSERADISH SAUCE

Horseradish is a classic condiment with beef. The sour cream mixture tames the bite of this pungently spicy root. Beef sirloin is an iron-rich protein source that is also rich in vitamin B12 and zinc.

Steak Ingredients:
1-pound sirloin steak, boneless, trimmed of excess fat
2 cloves garlic, cut in half
cooking spray
salt and pepper to taste

Sauce Ingredients:
1 clove garlic, minced
1/3 cup sour cream, fat-free
1½ tablespoons mayonnaise, reduced fat
1 tablespoon prepared white horseradish

Directions: Cut steak into four (4-ounce) pieces. Rub both sides of each steak with the cut garlic. Coat a 12-inch skillet with cooking spray and place over high heat until hot. Add steaks; cook 4 minutes. Turn steaks and cook 3 minutes longer so they have a good sear. Reduce heat to medium and cook to desired doneness. Season with salt and pepper to taste. For sauce, in a small bowl combine minced garlic, sour cream, mayonnaise, prepared white horseradish, salt, and pepper. Stir well and allow to rest at room temperature until serving. Nutrition: Serves 4 (1 steak and 2 tablespoons sauce). Per serving: 218 calories, 27 grams protein, 9 grams fat, 5 grams carbohydrate.

FLORENTINE T-BONE STEAK

I like to use T-bone steak, but any fat-marbled thick cut of beef will work nicely. Plan ahead as the marinating time is quite long and essential for the best results. One large steak serves four.

1 (16-ounce) T-bone steak
8 tablespoons extra virgin olive oil
4-5 fresh rosemary sprigs
3 cloves garlic, crushed
sea salt and freshly ground black pepper, to taste
balsamic vinegar and olive oil, to taste

Directions: Place the steak in a shallow dish. Mix together the olive oil, rosemary, garlic, salt, and pepper. Pour over the steak, cover and marinate in the refrigerator for 24 to 48-hours turning occasionally. Remove steak from refrigerator 30 minutes prior to cooking. Heat grill or broiler to high heat. Grill the meat over direct heat turning occasionally until desired doneness. Remove from grill and allow to rest 6 to 10 minutes. Drizzle steak with balsamic vinegar and olive oil. Slice steak crosswise against the grain in thin strips to serve. Nutrition: One 3-ounce serving of beef T-bone steak has 161 calories, 22 grams protein, 7 grams fat.

Beef Tenderloin Steaks with Red Pepper Sauce

Roasted red peppers bring a smoky flavor to this meal. Peppers are a super source of vitamin C and contain flavonoids that are believed to fight cancer. The sauce brings just enough moisture to the meat to aid chewing and digestion without it becoming a slider food.

4 (4-ounce) lean beef tenderloin steaks, boneless
1 tablespoon steak seasoning
salt to taste
1 teaspoon olive oil
1 (7-ounce) jar roasted red peppers in water, drained

Directions: Season each steak with steak seasoning and salt to taste. Heat the olive oil in a 10-inch skillet over medium-high heat. When hot cook steaks 4 to 6 minutes per side. While steaks cook place the roasted red peppers in a blender or food processor and blend until smooth. Season the sauce with salt and pepper to taste. Serve warm steaks with a drizzle of the red pepper sauce. Nutrition: Serves 4. Per serving: 188 calories, 25 grams protein, 3 grams carbohydrate.

DAY 6 RECIPES

Day 6 is the first day after the 5 Day Pouch Test and exemplifies how daily meals should be patterned to achieve the best results in weight loss and weight management after weight loss surgery. Every day is Day 6 which means meals are protein dense and nutritionally supported with complex carbohydrate in the form of vegetables, fruit, and scant servings of grains or starchy carbohydrates. Processed foods and simple sugars do not support our weight management objectives and should be avoided. Fat-saturated foods, such as deep fried food, should be avoided: high fat food does not support our health goals, adds excess non-nutritional calories to the diet, may lead to feelings of nausea and episodes of dumping syndrome (rapid gastric emptying), and ultimately lead to weight gain.

Historically as dieters we have placed great emphasis on counting calories. In the case of Day 6 it is more effective to practice "nutrient awareness" and follow a 2B/1B eating pattern eating two bites of protein for every one bite of complex carbohydrate–vegetable, fruit, or grain—and stop eating at the earliest signal of pouch fullness. This simple counting habit allows us to follow the "Protein First" rule.

Additionally, it relieves the burden of tracking calories and trying to meet traditional caloric intake recommendations that are not necessarily suited to the low volume meals required after restrictive bariatric surgery.

The following special section in this 5 Day Pouch Test Complete Recipe Collection includes 28 all new recipes that are examples of Day 6 meals to satiate our physical and mental hunger at the same time meeting our specific nutritional needs. You will also note a "Tested & Approved" badge on recipes that are suitable for inclusion in the 5DPT. The badge indicates which day of the plan to use the recipe.

Take a look at these new recipes and note how complex carbohydrates are included as ingredients to compliment the primary protein with texture and flavor, while also increasing the nutritional value of the food by providing vitamins and nutrients to cultivate improved nutritional health. Incidental dietary fats are part of each recipe and essential to vitamin and mineral absorption. It is widely accepted that healthy fats prolong feelings of satisfaction and prolong post-meal feelings of satiation which of course leads to less post-meal hunger and snacking.

Dietary fats: Keep in mind the important role of healthy monounsaturated fats as part of a balanced weight management diet. People who significantly lower or eliminate fat from their diet complain of constant distressing hunger. Research confirms they are not imagining this hunger. Fat consumed with abundant protein and complex carbohydrates slows the stomach from emptying: we feel full longer and nutrient absorption is increased. Healthy fats to include in your Day 6 diet are the monounsaturated fats found in olive, canola, and peanut oils as well as most nuts and avocados. Polyunsaturated fats are found in other plant-based oils, such as safflower, corn, sunflower, soybean, sesame, and cottonseed oils.

SMOOTHIES

Smoothies – icy beverages typically made with dairy and fruit ingredients and blended with ice – are a refreshing addition to the weight loss surgery high protein diet. The abundance of protein powder and protein drinks coupled with a varied selection of fresh and frozen fruit offers countless opportunities to enjoy the benefits of increased protein intake in a delicious nutrient-dense beverage. Use protein powder or ready to drink beverages that provide at least 15 grams of protein (whey protein isolate is the recommended protein by many bariatric nutritionists) and fewer than 5 grams of carbohydrate or sugar. Remember: Sugar is a simple carbohydrate and should only be included in the high protein diet in restricted moderation.

BLUEBERRY COCONUT SMOOTHIE

This tasty smoothie packs a protein and antioxidant punch while using one of my favorite new products, Silk® Vanilla Coconutmilk. This non-dairy "milk" adds a creamy, tropical taste to smoothies and pairs nicely with coffee. Each serving provides 50-percent more calcium than dairy milk and 90 calories per 1 cup serving. This product is free of dairy, soy, lactose, gluten, casein, egg and MSG and contains no artificial flavors or colors. Give it a try!

1 cup frozen blueberries

1 cup chilled Silk® Vanilla Coconutmilk

1-2 tablespoons maple syrup (or sweetener of choice)

1 scoop or single-serve packet vanilla whey protein powder

Directions: Reserve three or four blueberries for garnish. Combine all ingredients in a blender and blend until smooth. (May also be prepared in a shaker jar.) Serve immediately garnished with reserved blueberries. Nutrition will vary due to differences in protein powder. Blueberries are antioxidants and considered a super food. Flash-frozen berries are available year-round in your market's freezer section.

∗ *Shortcut: Blend 1 vanilla chilled Ready-to-Drink protein beverage with 1 cup frozen blueberries and 3 drops of coconut extract, adding ice as desired.*

New Products Shopping Hint

Routinely check your market for new products that are health and nutrition oriented. Most new products, such as the Silk® non-dairy milks, have website links that provide recipe and serving ideas using the products. This is a fun and dependable way to add new things to your menu without having to experiment your way to something tasty and satisfying. Also, check the Sunday newspaper advertising inserts for coupons and product ideas. Using coupons is a clever way to try new things at a lower cost on the grocery bill.

New Food Labels: January 2020 saw the introduction of new food labels as mandated by the FDA. The changes are intended to help us—

consumers—make better health choices. On packaging now look for serving size and calories in bolder type; an Added Sugars subset of carbohydrates; updated daily values, and overall reader-friendly appearance.

PUMPKIN SPICE HIGH PROTEIN LATTE

Enjoy this seasonal favorite while following your Protein First Day 6 diet. With about 24 grams of protein, the Pumpkin Spice Latte lets you indulge in the fantastic flavors of fall while staying on track.

1 cup hot freshly brewed coffee

1/2 cup 2% milk

¼ cup canned 100% pure pumpkin

1 scoop or single serve packet vanilla whey protein powder

1/4 teaspoon pumpkin or apple pie spice blend

1 packet sweetener of choice

Directions: Allow coffee to cool to below 130 degrees. To coffee add milk, pumpkin, vanilla whey protein powder, apple pie spice and sweetener in blender. Blend to combine, about 30 seconds. Serve immediately. One serving provides approximately 150 calories, 16-24 grams protein (depending on protein product used), 11 grams carbohydrate 2 grams fat.

✳   *Ingredient note: 2% milk may be substituted with lactose free milk, soymilk, rice milk, almond milk or other milk product of your choice.*

✳   *Spice Note: Apple Pie Spice Blend is a mixture of cinnamon, nutmeg, and allspice. Pumpkin Pie Spice Blend contains nutmeg, cloves, ginger, and cinnamon. Both are enticing additions to pumpkin based smoothies.*

EGGS - THE PERFECT PROTEIN

As we discussed in the Day 3 section (page 35) eggs are versatile, protein-packed staples that cook up into a perfect meal any time of year. Eating eggs might give your meal more staying power too. A recent study found that when people ate a scrambled-egg-and-toast breakfast, they felt more satisfied-and ate less at lunch-than when they ate a bagel (that supplied the same number of calories) another day. The combination of high protein and moderate fat in eggs might make them especially filling, say experts. Even if you're watching your cholesterol, a daily egg can likely fit into your eating plans.

For dozens more terrific egg recipes check out Volume 4 of our LivingAfterWLS Shorts: Breakfast Basics of WLS. Available in print and eBook updated for 2020.

SCRAMBLED EGG BURRITOS

These zesty Southwestern egg burritos are always a hit whether you serve them for breakfast, brunch, lunch or a casual dinner. The homemade black bean salsa adds a special touch, but these are extra-quick if you use your favorite jarred salsa.

4 (9-inch) whole-wheat flour tortillas
4 large eggs
1/8 teaspoon salt
freshly ground pepper, to taste
1 teaspoon extra-virgin olive oil
1 (4-ounce) can chopped green chilies
1/2 cup grated Cheddar, or pepper Jack cheese

2 cups Black Bean & Tomato Salsa (recipe follows) or prepared salsa
1/4 cup reduced-fat sour cream

Directions: Heat oven to 350°F. Wrap tortillas in foil and heat in the oven for 5 to 10 minutes. Whisk eggs, salt and pepper in a medium bowl with a fork until blended. Heat oil in a 10-inch nonstick skillet over medium-low heat. Add chilies and cook, stirring, for 1 minute. Add eggs and cook, stirring slowly with a wooden spoon or heatproof rubber spatula, until soft, fluffy curds form, 2 to 3 minutes. To serve, divide eggs evenly among the tortillas. Sprinkle each with 2 tablespoons cheese and roll up. Serve with salsa and sour cream on the side. Nutrition Serves 4. Per serving: 328 calories; 18 grams protein, 6 grams fat, 34 grams carbohydrate.

✳ *Black Bean & Tomato Salsa: Combine 1 can (14.5-ounces) drained and rinsed black beans with 1 cup prepared tomato-base salsa. Serve at room temperature; refrigerate remaining salsa.*

SMOKED SALMON & EGGS BENEDICT

I love traditional Eggs Benedict, but it can be a real pain to prepare and it is high in cholesterol and fat. This mock make-ahead eggs Benedict casserole delivers the great flavors we love without the hassle or the dietary guilt.

1 (0.9-ounce) envelope hollandaise sauce mix to make about 1 1/4 cup sauce
2 tablespoons capers drained
1/2 teaspoon finely shredded lemon peel
6 eggs

1/4 cup milk

1/8 teaspoon pepper

2 tablespoons margarine or butter

3 English muffins, split and toasted

6 ounces thinly sliced smoked salmon or Canadian-style bacon

1/4 cup soft breadcrumbs

1/2 cup shredded Parmesan cheese

Directions: For sauce, prepare hollandaise sauce mix according to package directions. Stir in the capers and lemon peel. Cover and set aside. In a medium bowl beat together eggs, milk, and pepper. In a large skillet melt 1 tablespoon of the margarine over medium heat. Pour in egg mixture. Cook, without stirring, until mixture begins to set on bottom and around edge. Using a spatula or a large spoon, lift and fold the partially cooked eggs so the uncooked portion flows underneath. Continue cooking for 3 to 4 minutes until eggs are cooked through but are still glossy and moist. Spread about 1/2 cup of the sauce over bottom of a 2-quart rectangular baking dish.

Arrange muffins, cut sides up, on top of sauce in dish. Divide smoked salmon or Canadian-style bacon into 6 equal portions. Place one portion, folded as necessary, on each muffin half. Spoon eggs onto muffin stacks, dividing evenly Spoon remaining sauce over eggs. For crumb topping, melt remaining margarine. Add breadcrumbs and grated Parmesan, tossing lightly to coat. Sprinkle over muffin stacks. Cover casserole and refrigerate up to 24 hours. One hour before serving remove from refrigerator. Heat oven to 350ºF. Bake casserole covered tightly with foil for 25 minutes or until heated through. If desired garnish with snipped fresh chives. Serve warm.

Nutrition: Serves 6. Per serving: 243 calories, 14 grams protein, 11 grams fat, 20 grams carbohydrate.

LIBBY'S BEST CREAMY PUMPKIN SOUP

Shared with permission from Very Best Baking by Nestle.

Vitamin Rich and Delicious: "Creamy Pumpkin Soup makes a great first course for a Thanksgiving meal or fall and winter entertaining," explains Libby's nutrition experts. Pumpkin is rich in vitamin A and a single serving of this soup provide 220% of the Recommended Daily Value.

1/4 cup (1/2 stick) butter or margarine
1 small onion, chopped
1 clove garlic, finely chopped
2 teaspoons packed brown sugar
1 can (14.5 fluid ounces) chicken broth
1/2 cup water
1/2 teaspoon salt (optional)
1/4 teaspoon ground black pepper
1 can (15 ounces) LIBBY'S® 100% Pure Pumpkin
1 can (12 fluid ounces) NESTLÉ® CARNATION® evaporated milk
1/8 teaspoon ground cinnamon

Directions: Melt butter in large saucepan over medium heat. Add onion, garlic and sugar; cook for 1 to 2 minutes or until soft. Add broth, water, salt and pepper; bring to a boil, stirring occasionally. Reduce heat to low; cook, stirring occasionally, for 15 minutes. Stir in pumpkin, evaporated milk and cinnamon. Cook, stirring occasionally, for 5 minutes. Remove from heat. Transfer mixture to food processor or blender (in batches, if necessary); process until smooth. Alternatively, use an immersion blender to puree mixture. Return to saucepan. Serve warm. Nutrition: Approximately five 1-cup servings. Per Serving: 230 calories, 7 grams protein, 15 grams fat (10 grams saturated) 17 grams carbohydrate, 4 grams dietary fiber.

CREAMY PUMPKIN SOUP CHANGE-UPS

For variety try these lip-smacking changeups to the basic creamy pumpkin soup recipe.

Chicken-Pumpkin Soup: Add 2 cups cooked shredded chicken to soup for last 5 minutes of cooking. Rotisserie chicken works wonderfully in this soup to boost the protein value.

Tex-Mex Vegetarian Pumpkin Soup: Add 1 can black beans, rinsed and drained; 1 (14.5-ounce) can southwestern style diced tomatoes; 1 cup shredded Cheddar cheese; 6 green onions, chopped, 1/2 cup sour cream. Add the beans and tomatoes at the same time you add the broth. Cook and stir as directed. Do not process with blender, keep the texture chunky. Ladle soup into bowls, top with cheese, green onions, and sour cream.

Bacon-Pumpkin Soup: Begin by cooking 1/2 pound of chopped bacon, 1 chopped yellow onion, and one clove minced garlic in soup pot over medium-high heat. When bacon is cooked and onions translucent remove 1/4 cup and set aside for garnish. Omit butter and proceed with basic recipe as directed. Serve warm, garnish with shredded Cheddar.

Apple-Pumpkin Soup: To increase sweetness add 1/3 cup apple juice to the soup mixture. Or add one small chopped apple to mixture for sweetness and extra fiber. Remove from heat and stir-in ½ cup low-fat cream cheese or Ricotta cheese.

Honey-Mustard Pumpkin Soup: Using the Basic Pumpkin Soup recipe omit the Splenda and crushed red pepper. Add 2 tablespoons honey and 1 tablespoon of prepared mustard.

Mushroom Pumpkin Soup: In a 2-quart saucepot sauté 1/2-cup of chopped yellow onion and 8 ounces sliced mushrooms. Season with salt and pepper, add the Basic Pumpkin Soup. Bring mixture to a low simmer and heat five minutes. Season with ground nutmeg.

COMFORT EATING IS OKAY IF....

From the moment we were born food has provided comfort to us. It is natural that we are compelled to reach for food when seeking comfort. This is not a character flaw: this is the human condition. Weight loss surgery does not take away our intrinsic human need to be comforted with nourishment. WLS gives us a second chance to rethink the type of nourishment we reach for when seeking comfort. Gone are the days of empty calorie comfort snacking. We are better nurtured with a warm cup of soup or a delicious meal of perfectly cooked protein and vegetables. Sweet berries or fruit provide far more sustenance and comfort than convenience store snacks and they come without the post-noshing guilt. I say, indeed, lets indulge in comforting by making wise nutritional decisions in response to the very real need. The desired result of comforting is to elevate mood and promote feelings of well-being. This is certain to happen when we make wise nutritional decisions and treat ourselves with kindness.

I strongly believe that the more we acknowledge rather than deny our need for comfort with nourishment, the more empowered we are to make healthful dietary choices.

Slow Cooker Turkey Chili

Early in the day prepare the chili and cook on low in a 3-quart slow cooker. When darkness falls serve up a bowl of robust turkey chili and let the comforting begin! Consider doubling the recipe and serve from a slow cooker at your next tailgate party for a guaranteed win.

1-pound lean ground turkey (white meat)
1 medium bell pepper finely chopped
1 small red onion, finely chopped
1 clove garlic, minced
2 cans (14 ounces) diced tomatoes, undrained
1 (16-ounce) can kidney beans, rinsed and drained
1 (15-ounce) can black beans, rinsed and drained
1 (14.5-ounce) can chicken or vegetable broth
1 (6-ounce) can tomato paste
1 tablespoon chili powder (mild or hot to taste)
1 tablespoon all-purpose seasoning blend

Optional Toppings: reduced-fat sour cream, plain yogurt, shredded cheese, minced fresh herbs.

Directions: In a large nonstick skillet, cook the ground turkey, bell pepper, red onion and garlic until meat is no longer pink. Drain. Transfer to a 4-quart slow cooker. In slow cooker stir in the tomatoes, kidney beans, black beans, broth, tomato paste, chili powder and seasoning. Cover and set to low. Cook for 6-8 hours. (Always follow the manufacturer's instructions provided with your slow cooker.) Serve warm with optional garnishes, as desired. Nutrition:

Approximately six 1-cup servings. Per serving: 210 calories, 29 grams protein, 3 grams fat, 24 grams carbohydrate, 8 grams dietary fiber.

CHICKEN & WHITE BEAN SOUP

Rotisserie chickens can really relieve the dinner-rush pressure-especially in this Italian-inspired soup that is quick to prepare.

2 teaspoons extra-virgin olive oil
2 leeks, white and light green parts only, chopped
1/4 teaspoon dried sage
2 (14-ounce) cans reduced sodium chicken broth
2 cups water
1 (15-ounce) can cannellini beans, rinsed and drained
4 cups shredded roasted rotisserie chicken

Directions: Heat oil in a Dutch oven over medium-high heat. Add leeks and cook, stirring often, until soft, about 3 minutes. Stir in sage and continue cooking until aromatic, about 30 seconds. Stir in broth and water, increase heat to high, cover and bring to a boil. Add beans and chicken and cook, uncovered, stirring occasionally, until heated through, about 10 minutes. Serve hot. Nutrition: Makes six 1½-cup servings. Per serving: 172 calories, 24 grams protein, 4 grams fat, 10 grams carbohydrate.

SALADS WITH PROTEIN

Debunk the myth that after weight loss surgery salad is not allowed. Do this by building a purposeful meal by assembling fresh ingredients and lean protein dressed in healthy fat. When carefully composed, such as these examples, a salad is well-suited to our high protein diet.

TUNA, SPINACH, AND STRAWBERRY SALAD

This salad is perfect any time of year. You can build it at the salad bar in your supermarket and simply add one pouch of water pack tuna for a tasty and filling lunch.

1-2 cups baby spinach or baby spring greens blend
1 cup sliced strawberries
1 tablespoon cheese of choice (feta is very good!)
1 tablespoon vinaigrette dressing
1 hard-cooked egg, crumbled
1 (2.6-ounce) package Starkist® Low Sodium Chunk Light Tuna

Directions: Toss all ingredients immediately prior to serving. Nutrition: Serves 1 providing 315 calories, 29 grams protein, 11 grams fat, 17 grams carbohydrate.

✳ *Ingredient Hint: Change-out the tuna for different protein including deli-style turkey or beef, shrimp, sliced steak, shredded chicken. The salad is a suitable foundation to enhance any cold-serve protein.*

TOMATO, BASIL AND FETA SALAD

This is a summer tomato salad that puts the best of the season on the plate. Other seasonal vegetables may be added such as steamed asparagus tips or green beans, sliced mushrooms or chopped avocado. To increase protein, add with grilled shrimp or chicken.

Salad Ingredients:
5 medium tomatoes, thinly sliced
1 medium red onion, thinly sliced
1 (6-ounce) package crumbled feta with dried basil and tomato
1 (2.25 ounce) can sliced ripe olives, drained

Dressing Ingredients:
1/2 cup olive oil
1/4 cup red wine vinegar
2 tablespoons chopped fresh basil
Fresh basil Leaves for garnish

Directions: Shortly before serving arrange the tomatoes and onion slices on a large serving platter. Top with the feta cheese and olives. In a jar with a tight-fitting lid, combine the oil, vinegar and basil; shake well. Drizzle over salad. Garnish with fresh basil leave. Nutrition: Serves 8. Per serving: 209 calories, 4 grams protein, 19 grams fat, 7 grams carbohydrate.

A WELL-DRESSED SALAD

Avoid using fat free dressings; they do not contribute nutritional value. Studies show that healthy monounsaturated fat, such as olive oil, is necessary for the absorption of vitamins and minerals. To promote the absorption of nutrients from fresh salad ingredients include a dressing made with olive oil. Consider a simple olive oil and balsamic vinegar dressing – a vinaigrette – to support good health, aid nutrient absorption, and improve digestion.

GRILLED CHICKEN & RASPBERRY SALAD

This refreshing salad can be prepared in less than 30 minutes. In a pinch use shredded rotisserie chicken fresh from the deli or leftover from a previous meal. Each serving provides 23 grams protein and 8 grams quality complex carbohydrates.

Dressing Ingredients:

1/4 cup raspberry vinegar
3 tablespoons canola oil
1/2 teaspoon poppy seeds
1/4 teaspoon salt
1/4 teaspoon black pepper

Grilled Chicken Ingredients:
1-pound skinless, boneless chicken breast halves
6 cups mixed salad greens
1/2 of a small red onion, thinly sliced and separated into rings
1 cup raspberries

Directions: For dressing, in a screw-top jar combine raspberry vinegar, oil, poppy seeds, salt and pepper. Cover and shake well. Set aside. Place chicken on the rack of an uncovered grill directly over medium coals. Grill for 12 to 15 minutes or until chicken is tender and no longer pink, turning once halfway through grilling. Place salad greens and onion on a large serving platter. Thinly slice chicken diagonally; arrange on top of greens mixture. Drizzle with dressing and top with fresh raspberries. Nutrition: Serves 4. Per serving: 255 calories, 23 grams protein, 8 grams carbohydrate, 14 grams fat.

CHICKEN CUTLETS AND CITRUS

Add citrus to savory chicken dishes for a satisfying and nutritious meal that keeps after-dinner cravings away.

LEMONY CHICKEN SALTIMBOCCA

Have you included citrus in your post-WLS menu? I find that when I enjoy a main dish that includes citrus the sweet-tart flavors help prevent post-meal cravings. This Lemony Chicken Saltimbocca is a classic poultry-citrus recipe for good reason: it's scrumptious. Serve orange slices on the side for added vitamins and flavor.

4 (4-ounce) chicken cutlets
1/8 teaspoon salt
12 fresh sage leaves
2 ounces very thinly sliced prosciutto, cut into 8 thin strips
(substitute thin-sliced bacon if prosciutto is unavailable)
4 teaspoons extra-virgin olive oil, divided
1/3 cup reduced sodium chicken broth
1/4 cup fresh lemon juice
1/2 teaspoon cornstarch
Lemon wedges (optional)

Directions: Sprinkle the chicken evenly with salt. Place 3 sage leaves on each cutlet; wrap 2 prosciutto slices around each cutlet, securing sage leaves in place. Heat a large skillet over medium heat. Add 1 tablespoon oil to pan, and swirl to coat. Add chicken to pan; cook for 2 minutes on each side or until done. Remove chicken from pan; keep warm. Combine broth, lemon juice, and cornstarch in a small bowl; stir with a whisk until smooth. Add cornstarch mixture and the remaining 1 teaspoon olive oil to pan; bring to a boil, stirring constantly. Cook for 1 minute or until slightly thickened, stirring constantly with a whisk. Spoon sauce over chicken and garnish with lemon wedges. Nutrition: Serves 4. Each serving of 1 cutlet and 2 tablespoons sauce provides: 202 calories, 30 grams protein, 8 grams fat, 3 grams carbohydrate.

SKILLET MARMALADE CHICKEN

Orange marmalade and freshly grated orange zest make a deliciously tangy sauce for quick-cooking chicken cutlets or chicken tenders. Try to use no-sugar added marmalade which is sweetened by naturally occurring sugars. Because the sugar content is very low per serving it is unlikely to cause dumping syndrome for gastric bypass patients. Sweet and savory main dishes help prevent hunger pangs and cravings. Avoid using artificially sweetened marmalade which may develop an unpleasant taste when cooked.

    Juice and zest from 1 orange
    2 tablespoons no-sugar added orange marmalade
    1 cup reduced sodium chicken broth
    2 tablespoons red-wine vinegar
    1 teaspoon Dijon-style mustard
    1 teaspoon cornstarch
    1-pound chicken cutlets or chicken tenders
    1/2 teaspoon kosher salt
    1/4 teaspoon freshly ground pepper
    6 teaspoons extra-virgin olive oil, divided
    2 large shallots, chopped

Directions: Zest orange, reserve. In a medium bowl juice orange. Add marmalade, broth, vinegar, mustard and cornstarch; whisk to blend. Season chicken cutlets with salt and pepper. Heat 4 teaspoons oil in a large skillet over medium-high heat. Add the chicken and cook until golden, about 2 minutes per side. Transfer to a plate and cover with foil to keep warm. Add the remaining 2 teaspoons oil and shallots to the pan and cook, stirring often, until golden and translucent, about 4 minutes. Add the marmalade mixture, gently simmer, whisking to lift the flavorful browned bits, until sauce is slightly reduced and thickened, about 2 minutes. Return chicken to skillet, toss with sauce and continue to simmer until chicken is heated through. Remove from the heat and stir in orange zest. Nutrition: Serves 4. Per serving: 213 calories; 24 grams protein, 8 grams fat, 10 grams carbohydrate.

SPEEDY TURKEY MELTS

Heat broiler. For each person place one low-carb whole grain tortilla on a baking sheet. Spread each tortilla with 1 tablespoon cranberry sauce or grape jelly; top with 3 ounces thinly sliced turkey (deli or roasted turkey) and 1 ounce sliced or shredded provolone cheese. Place under broiler and cook until bubbly and hot. Cut tortillas into fourths and serve warm with additional cranberry sauce or jelly. Refrigerate leftovers and enjoy for lunch or a mid-day protein break the next day. Each turkey melt provides 245 calories, 21 grams protein, 7 grams fat, 18 grams carbohydrate.

GRILLED PEPPERED PORK CHOPS WITH RELISH

This is showy and delicious and quite easy to prepare. The flavors are fresh and unusual making this a great weeknight company meal or good anytime meal to support a healthy and balanced diet.

6 (4 ounces each) boneless pork chops, 3/4-inch thick
1 (6-ounce) jar marinated artichoke hearts
1 teaspoon hot pepper sauce
1 1/2 cups diced tomatoes
1/2 cup chopped bottled roasted sweet red peppers
1/4 cup sliced ripe olives
1 small jalapeño pepper, seeded and finely chopped

Directions: Drain artichoke hearts, reserving liquid, add hot pepper sauce to the liquid. Place pork chops in a shallow baking dish, pour the pepper sauce mixture over chops and turn to coat. Let stand at room temperature for 30 minutes, turning chops occasionally. Drain chops, discarding marinade. While chops marinate prepare relish: chop artichoke hearts and combine with tomatoes, red peppers, olives, and jalapeño. Set aside. Prepare the grill or broiler to medium-high direct heat. Cook for 4 to 5 minutes each side until done (internal temperature 145ºF). Serve the relish with pork chops. Nutrition: Serves 6. Per serving of 1 chop and 2 tablespoons relish: 175 calories; 22 grams protein; 7 grams fat, 5 grams carbohydrate.

HERBED PORK CHOPS

This recipe is particularly protein dense and lean on fat. Enjoy it with fresh sliced tomatoes or lightly steamed summer squash or green beans. To feed a large group purchase a large pork tenderloin from the big box store and cut your own.

4 (4-ounce) center cut pork chops
1/2 teaspoon dried marjoram leaves
1/4 teaspoon garlic salt
1/4 teaspoon onion powder
1/8 teaspoon freshly ground black pepper
1 cup vegetable or chicken broth
1 tablespoon cornstarch mixed with 1 tablespoon cold water
2 tablespoons chopped parsley

Directions: Spray 12-inch nonstick skillet with cooking spray; heat over medium heat. Add pork chops and cook 10 minutes or until slightly browned, turning once. Combine marjoram, garlic salt, onion powder and pepper, season pork. Add 1/2 cup water to skillet; cover, reduce heat and cook 20 minutes or until pork reaches an internal temperature of 145ºF. Remove chops to plate and keep warm. Add cornstarch paste to pan juices; cook until thickened stirring constantly. Pour sauce over chops and garnish with parsley. Nutrition: Serves 4. Per serving: 169 calories; 19 grams protein, 10 grams fat 2 grams carbohydrate.

COMPLEX-CARB SIDE DISHES

Vegetables, fruit, and whole grains make fine side dishes to a high protein entrée. When thoughtfully prepared the addition of these complex carbohydrates enhance the meal both nutritionally and emotionally. Here are some ideas to inspire your creativity on the sides.

CHEESY BACON & TOMATO TOPPED POTATO SKINS

These bacon and tomato potato skins are a good way for weight loss surgery patients to enjoy potatoes without suffering from starch overload. Discard the insides of the potatoes or reserve them for another use. This recipe makes 24 potato wedges, each wedge is one serving.

6 large baking potatoes
2 teaspoons canola oil
1 teaspoon chili powder
1/2 teaspoon hot pepper sauce
2 small tomatoes, seeded and finely chopped
2 tablespoons finely chopped green onion
6 slices bacon, cooked crisp, drained, crumbled
1 cup shredded Cheddar cheese

1/2 cup dairy sour cream (optional)

Prepare Potato Skins: Scrub potatoes and prick with a fork. Arrange on a microwave-safe plate and microwave, uncovered, on high power for 15 to 20 minutes or until almost tender. Or bake potatoes in a 425ºF oven for 25 to 30 minutes until firm tender. Cool. Halve each potato lengthwise. Scoop out the inside of each potato half, leaving about a 1/4-inch thick shell. In a small bowl combine the oil, chili powder, and hot pepper sauce. Using a pastry brush, brush the insides of the potato shells with the oil mixture. Cut the potato shells in half lengthwise to make potato quarters. Place the potato quarters on a baking sheet and cover with plastic wrap. Refrigerate until baking time.

Prepare Topping: Toss together tomatoes and green onions, season with salt and pepper to taste. Cover and store refrigerated. Store chopped bacon and shredded cheddar separately, refrigerated. Just before serving heat oven to 450ºF. Remove plastic wrap from baking sheet of potato skins. Top each potato quarter with the tomatoes and onions, crisp crumbled bacon, and shredded Cheddar. Bake for 12 to 15 minutes or until cheese is melted and potato quarters are heated through. Serve with sour cream. Nutrition per 1 potato wedge: 70 calories, 3 grams protein, 3 grams fat, 8 grams carbohydrate

TANGY APPLE COLESLAW

1 (12-ounce) package broccoli coleslaw

1 large apple, chopped

1/4 cup light mayonnaise

2 tablespoons brown sugar

2 teaspoons chopped fresh rosemary

1 teaspoon cider vinegar

Directions: Combine all ingredients in a large bowl and toss well. Cover and chill. Prior to serving sample the slaw and season with salt and pepper as needed. Nutrition: 8 servings, 1/3-cup each. Per serving: 79 calories, 2 grams protein, 2 grams fat, 13 grams carbohydrate.

QUICK VEGGIE SIDES

BROILED TOMATOES

2 large ripe tomatoes
2 tablespoons olive oil vinaigrette
2 teaspoons salt-free garlic & herb seasoning blend
2 tablespoons fresh Parmesan cheese, shredded
2 tablespoons Italian-seasoned breadcrumbs.

Directions: Preheat broiler. Cut each tomato into 4 slices; place tomato slices on a broiler pan. Drizzle with vinaigrette; season with salt-free garlic and herb seasoning blend. Combine cheese and breadcrumbs; sprinkle over tomato slices. Broil 3 to 5 minutes or until cheese melts. Nutrition: Serves 4, two tomato slices each. Per serving: 58 calories, 3 grams protein, 3 grams fat, 8 grams carbohydrate.

SUMMER SQUASH SKILLET:

Using a combination of zucchini and yellow squash cut in ¼-inch slices to measure about 4 cups. Heat 1 tablespoon olive oil in a medium skillet, add sliced squash, cook and stir until crisp-tender. Season with lemon zest, salt, and pepper. Serve warm.

HONEY GLAZED CARROTS

Cook an 8-ounce package of fresh sliced carrots with 1 tablespoon water in the microwave on high for 3 to 4 minutes until crisp-tender. Carefully drain and toss hot carrots with 1 tablespoon honey and 1 tablespoon yogurt "butter" spread. (See Ingredient Note page 56). Season with coarse salt and freshly ground pepper. Serve warm.

OVEN ROASTED ASPARAGUS

Clean 1-pound fresh asparagus snapping off and discarding woody stems and peeling outer skin with a vegetable peeler. (This makes asparagus easier for the WLS-patient to digest.) Toss prepared asparagus with 1-2 teaspoons olive oil and place on rimmed baking sheet. Bake in heated 450ºF oven 10 minutes until tender. Season with salt and pepper and serve warm.

EASY GREEN SALAD TOSS

In a large bowl toss together 8 cups prepared salad greens with ¼ cup ready-made vinaigrette and 1-ounce grated Parmesan cheese. Divide among four chilled salad plates and serve with toasted sunflower seeds and fresh seasonal berries.

RASPBERRY YOGURT PARFAITS

In dessert dishes or parfait glasses alternate layers of raspberries and yogurt for a refreshing snack or special occasion dessert. To make four servings use 2 cups of raspberries and 4 (5.3-ounce) cartons of single serving Chobani Simply 100 ® Vanilla Greek Yogurt and ¼-cup toasted almonds. Garnish with berries and toasted almonds. One serving provides 12 grams of protein for fewer than 150 calories.

KAYE BAILEY

Kaye Bailey developed the 5 Day Pouch Test in 2007 and is the owner of LivingAfterWLS and the 5 Day Pouch Test websites. Ms. Bailey, a professional research journalist, and a bariatric RNY (gastric bypass) patient since 1999, brings professional research methodology and personal experience to her publications focused on long-lasting successful weight management after surgery.

Concerned about weight regain her bariatric surgeon advised her to "get back to basics". With that vague advice Ms. Bailey says, "I read thousands of pages and conducted interviews with medical professionals including surgeons, nutritionists, and mental health providers. I collected data from WLS post-ops who honestly and generously shared their experience. My research background gave me the methodology to collect a vast amount of data. As a patient I found answers to the questions and concerns I have in common with most patients after WLS." From that the 5DPT and related works evolved.

Kaye Bailey is the author of countless articles syndicated in several languages, and books available in print and electronic format including:

The 5 Day Pouch Test Owner's Manual

Day 6: Beyond the 5 Day Pouch Test

Cooking with Kaye Methods to Meals: Protein First Recipes

5 Day Pouch Test Complete Recipe Collection

Protein First: Understanding & Living the First Rule of WLS.

See Kaye's author page for a current catalog of all our publications. Kaye Bailey Amazon Page

She serves as Executive Editor of the LivingAfterWLS Personal Solutions journals and planners available at Amazon and the LAWLS Bookstore. The Personal Solutions planners and journals are success promoting tools for people that believe healthy living should be a simple and painless way of life.

DAY 6: BEYOND THE 5 DAY POUCH TEST

BY KAYE BAILEY (2ND EDITION 2020)

This updated on-point 2nd Edition release of Kaye Bailey's acclaimed Day 6: Beyond the 5 Day Pouch Test (2009) positions you for your best healthy weight management life. Times have changed: the basics remain true. Advanced medical and scientific understanding of obesity paired with Kaye's real-world basics come together this powerful guidebook for epic WLS success. Kaye Bailey had gastric bypass in 1999 and has maintained her weight loss for 20 years. Don't you want to know her secrets?

* Lose more weight
* Maintain a healthy weight
* Steady your body chemistry & energy
* Uplift your confidence & improve mood
* Mind management after WLS
* Learn how to work the Four Rules of WLS
* Achieve your goals: Live your dreams

You have the ability to be successful with bariatric surgery. Learn to empower your inner strength through learning, experience, kindness, forgiveness, acceptance and gratitude. Exploit your inner potential and thrive in the life you deserve. Day 6 shows you how.

RECIPE INDEX

5 DAY POUCH TEST RECIPES   21
BEFORE YOU START: TAME A GRUMPY POUCH   22
FENNEL AND CELERY "GRUMPY POUCH" SOUP   22
WARM LEMON WATER   23

DAYS 1 & 2: LIQUIDS   25

CHOCO-MOCHA MORNING SMOOTHIE   26
VANILLA-BERRY SMOOTHIE   27
STRAWBERRIES & WHITE CHOCOLATE SMOOTHIE   27
HIGH PROTEIN PUDDING   28
FROZEN PROTEIN PUDDING POPS   28
HIGH PROTEIN GELATIN   29
HAM & CHEESE SOUP   31
LOW-CARB PUMPKIN & SAUSAGE SOUP   32
PUMPKIN SHRIMP SOUP   34
LEMONY CHICKEN SOUP   35
TOMATO-CHICKPEA SOUP: VEGETARIAN   37
CREAM OF TURKEY SOUP   41
HAM & SPLIT PEA SOUP   41
BLACK BEAN SOUP: VEGETARIAN   43
LENTIL & BARLEY SOUP: VEGETARIAN   44
HOT & SOUR SOUP: LACTO-OVO VEGETARIAN   45

DAY 3: SOFT PROTEIN   47

MOCHA PEANUT BUTTER BITES   48
HARD-COOKED EGGS   49
MOCK BREAKFAST BURRITO   50
BACON SWISS SQUARES   51
SPINACH-SAUSAGE EGG BAKE   52
EGG BRUNCH BAKE   53
PUFFY TURKEY & SWISS OMELET   54
TO-GO: CRANBERRY TURKEY ROLL-UPS   55
PARMESAN TUNA PATTIES   56

FISH CAKES 57
SALMON PATTIES 59
SALMON AND BLACK BEAN PATTIES 59

DAY 4: *FIRM PROTEIN* 63
HALIBUT WITH FETA-SPINACH TOPPING 64
SUNFLOWER ORANGE ROUGHY 65
SALMON WITH MUSTARD CREAM SAUCE 66
ORANGE GLAZED SALMON 67
TUNA STEAKS WITH SALSA & AVOCADO 67
SESAME TUNA 68
PARMESAN BAKED FISH 69
BUTTERY LEMON SHRIMP 70
SPICY STIR-FRY SHRIMP 71
CITRUS BAY SCALLOPS 72
PAN-SEARED SCALLOPS WITH CHERRY TOMATOES 73
SLOW COOKER THAI PEANUT MEATBALLS 74
TURKEY-PARMESAN-PESTO MEATBALLS 74
VEGGIE MUSHROOM-SWISS PATTY MELTS 75
CLASSIC SALISBURY STEAK 76

DAY 5: *SOLID PROTEIN* 79
CHIPOTLE-JALAPENO CHICKEN WITH BLACK BEANS 79
MUSTARD BAKED CHICKEN 80
PEPPER-LIME CHICKEN 81
CHICKEN WITH CANNELLINI BEANS 82
SLOW COOKER CHICKEN PARMESAN 82
CHICKEN AND EDIBLE POD PEAS 83
SLOW COOKER GARLIC & THYME CHICKEN THIGHS 84
TURKEY-AVOCADO-SWISS STACK 84
TURKEY TENDERLOIN WITH MUSTARD MUSHROOM SAUCE 85
SEARED PORK TENDERLOIN CHOPS WITH BALSAMIC SAUCE 86
SKILLET PORK CHOPS WITH HONEY-MUSTARD SAUCE 87
SIRLOIN STEAKS WITH HORSERADISH SAUCE 88
FLORENTINE T-BONE STEAK 89
BEEF TENDERLOIN STEAKS WITH RED PEPPER SAUCE 90

DAY 6 RECIPES	*91*
BLUEBERRY COCONUT SMOOTHIE	93
PUMPKIN SPICE HIGH PROTEIN LATTE	95
SCRAMBLED EGG BURRITOS	96
SMOKED SALMON & EGGS BENEDICT	97
LIBBY'S BEST CREAMY PUMPKIN SOUP	99
CREAMY PUMPKIN SOUP CHANGE-UPS	100
CHICKEN & WHITE BEAN SOUP	103
TUNA, SPINACH, AND STRAWBERRY SALAD	104
TOMATO, BASIL AND FETA SALAD	104
GRILLED CHICKEN & RASPBERRY SALAD	105
LEMONY CHICKEN SALTIMBOCCA	106
SKILLET MARMALADE CHICKEN	107
SPEEDY TURKEY MELTS	109
GRILLED PEPPERED PORK CHOPS WITH RELISH	109
HERBED PORK CHOPS	110
CHEESY BACON & TOMATO TOPPED POTATO SKINS	111
TANGY APPLE COLESLAW	112
BROILED TOMATOES	113
SUMMER SQUASH SKILLET:	113
HONEY GLAZED CARROTS	113
OVEN ROASTED ASPARAGUS	114
EASY GREEN SALAD TOSS	114
RASPBERRY YOGURT PARFAITS	114

A LIVINGAFTERWLS PUBLICATION

Kaye Bailey

Proudly serving the healthy weight management and weight loss surgery community since 2005.

Cover © LivingAfterWLS
Adobe Stock Licensed Image by Jenifoto
ISBN-13: 978-1518844201